Statistics at Square One

Statistics at Square One

T. D. V. Swinscow

Articles published in
the *British Medical Journal*

Published by the British Medical Association
Tavistock Square, London WC1H 9JP

First edition	1976
Second edition	1977
Reprinted June	1977
Reprinted Sept.	1977
Reprinted Nov.	1977
Third edition March	1978
Fourth edition October	1978
Reprinted Dec.	1978

Made and Printed in England by
Dawson & Goodall Ltd.
The Mendip Press, Bath.

Contents

Introduction

Many observations made in medicine are most naturally expressed in words. For instance, we might say, "His pulse could not be recorded." But for many others the most natural mode of expression is in numbers, as in the phrase, "His pulse was beating at 80 per minute." The purpose of statistical methods is to put numerical data into a context by which their meaning can be better judged. The intention of this book is to illustrate the use of such methods. No knowledge of mathematic beyond an elementary level is required. The examples are drawn mainly from clinical medicine but may be readily adapted to other branches of biology.

Some familiarity with statistical methods is advantageous—even essential—for two reasons. Firstly, just as discussing his data in words often helps an investigator to understand them better, so testing the numerical results statistically by his own effort gives him a clearer view of their significance. Secondly, statisticians themselves are busy if helpful people, and are not always available to solve the fairly simple problems discussed in this book.

For the analysis of medical and many other biological problems complicated statistical methods are rarely necessary. In contrast much ingenuity often has to be devoted to the plan of research so that the investigator may obtain truly comparable, complete, random samples. Thereafter the statistical analysis of them is best kept as simple as possible. In fact, data that fail to yield a significant result when subjected to simple tests but do so after a refined and complex analysis need to be looked at especially critically. Success here may be due to the use of more information by the complex method than the simple. But it may also depend on the existence of differences that have no practical importance. It is worth bearing in mind that statistical significance does not necessarily imply clinical significance. Thorough and detailed planning of an investigation is what should come first. After that a simple statistical analysis generally provides the most conclusive results for application in practice.

The small, moderately priced electronic calculators now generally available make the computation of elementary statistics an easy matter. The methods described here are therefore adapted to their use. Suitable instruments have keys for squares, square roots, change of sign, and a memory in addition to the usual arithmetical keys. Though simpler calculators can be of help, keys for squares and square roots save much

Introduction

labour, while a memory obviates the need to record intermediate stages of some calculations on paper. More complex (and more expensive) calculators with special statistical functions exist, but they are unnecessary for the calculations to be discussed here. One of the great advantages of the electronic over the older mechanical calculators is that they provide instant squares and square roots at the push of a button. A disadvantage of many electronic calculators is that they cannot handle numbers of more than eight digits. Methods of overcoming this limitation when computing the standard deviation are described in Chapter 13.

A practical point when choosing a calculator is that a model with rechargeable batteries is more convenient and economical than one with ordinary batteries, provided a main supply of electricity exists for the recharging.

For the third edition the chapter on the exact probability test has been partly rewritten to clarify the text.

This book is based on a series of articles, here revised and extended, which were published in the *British Medical Journal* in 1976. In its preparation I received invaluable advice from Professor P Armitage, for which I am most grateful. I am also grateful to the following readers of the articles who gave critical advice on them: Dr A W F Edwards, Dr I D Hill, Dr D Middleton, and Professor R G Record. The faults that remain are certainly mine.

1. Tabulation and mean

Before any statistical calculation, even of the simplest kind, is performed on data they are tabulated. If they are relatively few, say up to about 30, they are conveniently written down in order of size.

For example, Dr Green, a paediatric registrar in a district general hospital, is investigating the amount of lead in the urine of children from a nearby housing estate. In a particular street there are 15 children whose ages range from 1 year to under 16, and in a preliminary study he has found the following amounts of urinary lead (in μmol/24 h), taken from his notes in random order and then set down thus in what is sometimes called an *array*:

TABLE 1.1—*Urinary concentration of lead in 15 children, μmol/24*

0·1, 0·4, 0·6, 0·8, 1·1, 1·2, 1·3, 1·5, 1·7, 1·9, 1·9, 2·0, 2·2, 2·6, 3·2

The advantage of first setting the figures out in order of size and not simply feeding them straight from the notes into a calculator (for example, to find their mean) is that the relation of each to the next can be looked at. Is there a steady progression, a noteworthy hump, a considerable gap? Simple inspection can disclose irregularities. Furthermore, a glance at the figures gives information on their *range*. The smallest is 0·1 and the largest 3·2. To find their *mean* (or average) Dr Green adds them up, getting a total of 22·5, and divides this by the number of observations, 15, to get 1·5 μmol/24 h.

FREQUENCY DISTRIBUTION

But the results from only 15 children are too few for Dr Green's purpose, so he extends his inquiry to the whole of the small industrial estate in which the street lies. In consequence he obtains figures for the urinary lead concentration in 140 children aged over 1 year and under 16. To make them manageable these figures are best tabulated in a *frequency distribution*. This is simply a classification of numbers of children by the concentration of lead in their urine, so that against successive amounts of lead the corresponding number of children will be recorded.

To make this classification Dr Green must decide on suitable class boundaries for the lead concentrations in his frequency distribution. If the classes are too small the table will be unwieldy; if they are too large, information will be lost by being too summary. The divisions chosen must also be such that the actual data can easily be allotted to them, and they must be mutually exclusive.

The range of readings for the 140 children was 0·1 to 4·2 μmol/24 h. If the classes are set at intervals of 0·5 μmol/24 h, nine will be needed to cover this range; if at 0·4, 11; if at 0·25, 18; and if at 0·2, 22. Between about 10 and 20 classes are generally acceptable in practice. It is also helpful to fix the class intervals so that the half-way points between them are instantly evident on inspection, because they will be needed for calculation of the mean and standard deviation. Thus half way between 1·8 and 2·0 is clearly 1·9, but half way between 1·75 and 2·0 is not so immediately obvious (1·875). Finally, classes are better initially chosen to be too small than too large, because small ones can easily be amalgamated later to form large ones if necessary. Weighing up these somewhat conflicting considerations, Dr Green decided to start with class intervals of 0·2, providing 22 classes.

The tabulation of the data from notes is done as shown in fig 1.1, a stroke being placed for each value of lead concentration against its

Lead concentration (μmol/24h)			
0 –	I		I
0·2 –	I		I
0·4 –	III		3
0·6 –	IIII		4
0·8 –	++++		5
1·0 –	++++		5
1·2 –	++++ II		7
1·4 –	++++ IIII		9
1·6 –	++++ ++++ I		11
1·8 –	++++ ++++ II		12
2·0 –	++++ ++++ ++++		15
2·2 –	++++ ++++ III		13
2·4 –	++++ ++++		10
2·6 –	++++ IIII		9
2·8 –	++++ IIII		9
3·0 –	++++ II		7
3·2 –	++++		5
3·4 –	++++ I		6
3·6 –	III		3
3·8 –	IIII		4
4·0 –			0
4·2 –	I		1
4·4			0
Total			140

FIG 1.1—Tabulation of data to construct a frequency distribution

class interval. When four strokes have accumulated they are scored through with a fifth to facilitate counting in groups of five. Because the intervals of 0·2 μmol/24 h used in this first tabulation led to rather a large table Dr Green decided to compile a second table from it with class intervals of double the size—namely, 0·4 μmol/24 h. He felt free to do this because, firstly, the distribution of patients progresses fairly steadily from class to class, so that amalgamation will not obscure real discontinuities between classes; and, secondly, because the figures themselves are not so precise as they may appear to be, for they are subject to errors of physiological variation, clinical sampling, and laboratory measurement. The result of amalgamating the 0·2 μmol classes to form 0·4 μmol classes is shown in table 1.2. It includes the total number of children. But is it correct to base calculations on this total group of 140 ? Some problems there are discussed below (p 5).

TABLE 1.2—*Lead concentration in urine of children*

Lead concentration (μmol/24 h)	Number of children
0 –	2
0·4 –	7
0·8 –	10
1·2 –	16
1·6 –	23
2·0 –	28
2·4 –	19
2·8 –	16
3·2 –	11
3·6 –	7
4·0 –	1
4·4	
Total	140

In calculating the mean we add up the observed values and divide by the number of them. The total of the values obtained in Dr Green's first study was 22·5 μmol/24 h, which was divided by their number, 15, to give a mean of 1·5 μmol/24 h. This familiar process is conveniently expressed by the following symbols:

$$\bar{x} = (\Sigma x)/n.$$

$\bar{x}$ (pronounced x bar) signifies the mean; x is each of the values of urinary lead; n is the number of these values; and Σ, the Greek capital sigma, denotes "sum of".

MEAN FROM FREQUENCY DISTRIBUTION

When Dr Green extended his study and obtained the urinary lead concentrations from 140 children, he tabulated the findings as shown in the first two columns of table 1.3, which are the same as in table 1.2.

To calculate the mean of the 140 lead concentrations it is of course possible to add up individually the original results obtained in the laboratory and to divide them by 140. A less laborious method, and one that follows naturally from the tabulation of the results in a frequency distribution, is illustrated in table 1.3. Two assumptions are made. The first is that the lead concentrations can take any numerical value in the range, though the sensitivity of the apparatus used to measure them does in practice impose some limits on the continuity.

TABLE 1.3—*Calculation of mean lead concentration in urine of 140 children*

(1) Lead concentration μmol/24 h	(2) Number of children	(3) Midway points of col (1)	(4) Col (3) × col (2)
0 –	2	0·2	0·4
0·4 –	7	0·6	4·2
0·8 –	10	1·0	10·0
1·2 –	16	1·4	22·4
1·6 –	23	1·8	41·4
2·0 –	28	2·2	61·6
2·4 –	19	2·6	49·4
2·8 –	16	3·0	48·0
3·2 –	11	3·4	37·4
3·6 –	7	3·8	26·6
4·0 –	1	4·2	4·2
4·4			
Total	140		305·6

Mean lead concentration = 305·6/140 = 2·18 μmol/24 h.

(Continuous and discrete variables are discussed more fully below.) The second assumption is that the results within any given class interval (for example, the 7 results in the interval 0·4 up to 0·8) are distributed evenly along the interval. The midway point represents that interval better than points nearer its top or bottom. Thus 7 × 0·6 will, on the average, give a better estimate of the sum of those 7 results than 7 × 0·4 or 7 × 0·79 or 7 × any other number in between. For this reason the midway points of the class intervals are set out in col (3). In col (4) the value of each midway point is multiplied by the number of children in the class. The sum of the lead concentrations is then put at the bottom of col (4)—namely, 305·6. To find the mean lead concentration in the 140 specimens, this sum is divided by 140, giving 2·18 μmol/24 h.

If this procedure is carried out on a calculator with a memory, the figures in col (4) need not be written out. The multiplication of each value of lead concentration is done, the result added into the memory, and the sum extracted from the memory at the end. Further, if the class intervals in col (1) are carefully chosen, as recommended above (p 2), it may be possible (as it is here) to see the midway point by inspection. Col (3) is then superfluous, and the calculation can be done with the aid of the calculator straight from table 1.2 without the need for additional columns.

ADDING LIKE AND UNLIKE

The question was asked on p 3 whether it was correct to make calculations on the total group of 140 children. In so far as they are children, the sources of these observations clearly belong to the same class of creatures and have much in common. But as parents have often had occasion to remark, children differ greatly among themselves. Some are boys, some are girls, some (in this group) were near the age of 1 and others nearly 16. Disparities of this kind often lie hidden but need to be thought of.

For example, according to the Registrar General's estimate for mid-1973, the population of the Birmingham hospital region was 5,163,200 and that for the South-western hospital region 3,246,200. But women constituted 50·49% of the Birmingham region and 51·80% of the South-western, a difference of 1·31%. This might be large enough to invalidate a comparison between the incidence of a disease in the two regions if women were particularly susceptible or relatively immune to it. Furthermore, while 35% of people in the Birmingham region were aged 45 or over, the figure for the South-western region was 41%. Susceptibility to many diseases varies with age, so that this difference too must be taken account of in any comparison between the regions. The figures for the total populations of these two regions conceal important dissimilarities between them.

Likewise when studying the urinary lead concentrations it would be advisable to analyse them according to the age and sex of the children. It is possible, for instance, that the younger children, having less judgment of what is safe to put in their mouths, might have higher lead concentrations than the older children; and boys, being more exploratory than girls, might have got more lead-contaminated material from a forbidden site.

Exercise 1.1. In another group of children Dr Green found the following urinary lead concentrations (in μmol/24 h): 0·02, 0·24, 1·72, 2·98, 1·32, 0·95, 1·44, 3·12, 1·15, 0·87, 1·21, 2·02, 0·91, 2·03, 0·31, 0·52. What is the mean? *Answer:* 1·30.

Exercise 1.2. From the 140 children whose urinary concentration of lead he had investigated Dr Green selected the 40 who were aged at least 1 year but under 5. He found in the urine the following concentrations of copper in μmol/24 h:

0·70,	0·45,	0·72,	0·30,	1·16,	0·69,	0·83,	0·74,
1·24,	0·77,	0·65,	0·76,	0·42,	0·94,	0·36,	0·98,
0·64,	0·90,	0·63,	0·55,	0·78,	0·10,	0·52,	0·42,
0·58,	0·62,	1·12.	0·86,	0·74,	1·04,	0·65,	0·66,
0·81,	0·48,	0·85,	0·75,	0·73,	0·50,	0·34,	0·88,

What is the mean when calculated (1) from the individual observations, (2) from a frequency distribution of the observations arranged at intervals of 0·1 from 0·1 to 1·3 μmol/24 h? *Answer:* (1) 0·6965, (2) 0·705 μmol/24 h.

2. Standard deviation

In addition to knowing the mean value of a series of measurements it is often informative to have some idea of their range about the mean. For example, the measurements of the urinary concentration of lead that Dr Green obtained for 15 children ranged from 0·1 to 3·2 μmol/24 h, with a mean of 1·5. When he extended his study to 140 children the range was from 0·1 to 4·2, with a mean of 2·18 μmol/24 h.

The range is an important measurement, for the figures at the top and bottom of it denote the findings furthest removed from the generality. However, they do not give much indication of the spread of the observations about the mean. This is where the standard deviation comes in.

The theoretical basis of the standard deviation is complex and need not trouble the ordinary user of it. But a practical point to note is that, whether the calculation is done on the whole "population" of data or on a sample drawn from it, the population itself should at least approximately fall into a so-called "normal" (or Gaussian) distribution. When it does so the standard deviation provides a useful basis for interpreting the data in terms of probability. (Some discussion of "populations" and "samples" appears on p 16.)

The normal distribution is represented by a family of curves, not a single, unique curve. It expresses a certain relationship between the mean and the square of the standard deviation (variance). The curves are always symmetrically bell-shaped, but the extent to which the bell is compressed or flattened out depends on the variance of the population. However, the mere fact that a curve is bell-shaped does not mean that it represents a normal distribution, since other distributions may have that sort of shape.

Many biological characteristics conform to a normal distribution closely enough for it to be commonly used—for example, heights of adult men and women, blood pressures in a healthy population, random errors in many types of laboratory measurements and of biochemical data. Fig 2.1 shows a normal curve calculated from the diastolic blood pressures of 500 men, mean 82 mm Hg, standard deviation 10 mm Hg. The ranges representing ±1 SD, ±2 SD, and ±3 SD about the mean are marked.

The reason why the standard deviation is such a useful measure of the scatter of the observations is this: if the observations follow a "normal" distribution, a range covered by one standard deviation above the mean and one standard deviation below it ($\bar{x} \pm 1$ SD) includes about 68% of the observations, a range of 2 standard deviations

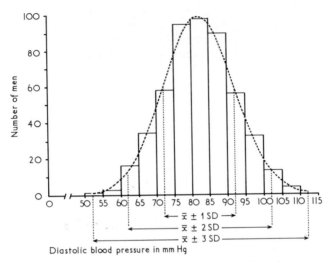

FIG 2.1—Normal curve calculated from diastolic blood pressures of 500 men, mean 82 mm Hg, standard deviation 10 mm Hg.

above and 2 below ($\bar{x} \pm 2$ SD) about 95% of the observations, and of 3 standard deviations above and 3 below ($\bar{x} \pm 3$ SD) about 99·73% of the observations. Consequently if we know the mean and standard deviation of a set of observations, we can obtain some useful information by simple arithmetic. By putting 1, 2, or 3 standard deviations above and below the mean we can estimate the ranges that would be expected to include about 68%, 95%, and 99·7% of the observations.

STANDARD DEVIATION FROM UNGROUPED DATA

The standard deviation is a summary measure of the differences of each observation from the mean. If the differences themselves were added up, the positive would exactly balance the negative and so their sum would be 0. Consequently the squares of the differences are added. The sum of the squares is then divided by the number of observations minus one to give the mean of the squares, and the square root is taken to bring the measurements back to the units we started with. (The division by the number of observations *minus one* instead of the number of observations itself to obtain the mean square is because "degrees of freedom" must be used. In these circumstances they are one less than the total. The theoretical justification for this need not trouble the user in practice.)

This procedure is now illustrated from table 2.1 with the 15 readings obtained by Dr Green in his preliminary study of urinary lead concentrations. The readings are set out in col (1). In col (2) is recorded the difference between each reading and the mean. The sum of the differences is 0. In col (3) the differences are squared, and the sum of those squares is at the bottom of the column.

TABLE 2.1—*Calculation of standard deviation*

(1) Lead concentration, μmol/24 h x	(2) Differences from mean $x - \bar{x}$	(3) Differences squared $(x - \bar{x})^2$	(4) Observations in col (1) squared x^2
0·1	− 1·4	1·96	0·01
0·4	− 1·1	1·21	0·16
0·6	− 0·9	0·81	0·36
0·8	− 0·7	0·49	0·64
1·1	− 0·4	0·16	1·21
1·2	− 0·3	0·09	1·44
1·3	− 0·2	0·04	1·69
1·5	0	0	2·25
1·7	0·2	0·04	2·89
1·9	0·4	0·16	3·61
1·9	0·4	0·16	3·61
2·0	0·5	0·25	4·00
2·2	0·7	0·49	4·84
2·6	1·1	1·21	6·76
3·2	1·7	2·89	10·24
Total 22·5	0	9·96	43·71

n = 15, $\bar{x} = 1·5$.

The sum of the squares of the differences (or deviations) from the mean, 9·96, is now divided by the total number of observations minus one, to give the *variance*. Thus, the variance =

$$\frac{\Sigma(x-\bar{x})^2}{n-1}.$$

Finally, the square root of the variance provides the standard deviation:

$$SD = \sqrt{\frac{\Sigma(x-\bar{x})^2}{n-1}}.$$

This procedure illustrates the structure of the standard deviation, but in practice it is calculated less laboriously. Finding all the deviations

of the observations from the mean, as in table 2.1, col (2), can be
bypassed.

If the number of observations is not too many—say, up to 100—
they are set out in one or more columns as shown in table 2.1, col (1).
Their sum is put at the bottom and their mean calculated as before.
Each observation is then squared, as shown in table 2.1, col (4), and the
sum of the squares set down ($= 43.71$). We now square the sum of the
observations (foot of col (1)), divide that by the number of observations,
and subtract the result from the sum of the squares of the observations
(foot of col (4)). Dr Green's figures are treated as follows:

$$43.71 - \frac{22.5^2}{15}. \text{ This equals } 9.96.$$

The figure thus obtained is the same as the 9.96 at the foot of the
table 2.1, col (3). The reason for this is that

$$\Sigma x^2 - \frac{(\Sigma x)^2}{n} = \Sigma(x - \bar{x})^2.$$

We now find the variance by dividing 9.96 by 14 (which is $n - 1$), and
so obtain 0.714. The square root of this is the standard deviation, 0.84.

The procedure may be summarised as follows:

Tabulate the observed figures in a column
and add them   ..   .. Σx

Square this total   ..   .. $(\Sigma x)^2$

Divide by the number of observations   .. $\dfrac{(\Sigma x)^2}{n}$ (1)

Square each observed figure ..   .. x^2

Add the squares   ..   .. Σx^2 (2)

Subtract (1) from (2)   ..   .. $\Sigma x^2 - \dfrac{(\Sigma x)^2}{n}$

Divide by the number of observations minus one   .. $\dfrac{\Sigma x^2 - \dfrac{(\Sigma x)^2}{n}}{n - 1}$

Take the square root   ..   .. $\sqrt{\dfrac{\Sigma x^2 - \dfrac{(\Sigma x)^2}{n}}{n - 1}}$

This is the standard deviation

A calculator with a memory and keys for squares and square roots
makes light work of this procedure. All that need be set on paper is
the column of figures. Each is squared in turn on the calculator, and

the squares are accumulated in the memory. The sum of the figures is then added up on the calculator, squared, and divided by the number of observations. This total is subtracted from the sum of squares in the memory. The resulting difference is extracted from the memory on to the display screen, and divided by the number of observations minus one. The square root then gives the standard deviation.

STANDARD DEVIATION FROM GROUPED DATA

Often the standard deviation must be calculated on such a large number of data that they need to be grouped for convenient handling. We have already met this necessity with the calculation of the mean. When Dr Green had only 15 readings for concentration of lead in the urine he could keep them separate in an array. But when he collected 140 readings he compiled a frequency distribution to make them manageable (table 1.2).

The calculation of the standard deviation from data grouped in a frequency distribution is similar to the calculation from ungrouped data, but one important point needs watching. As with the calculation of the mean from grouped data, the *midpoint* in each class is taken as the reading.

TABLE 2.2—*Calculation of standard deviation from grouped data (continuous variable)*

(1) Lead concentration μmol/24 h	(2) Number of children	(3) Midpoints of col (1)	(4) Col (2) × col (3)	(5) Midpoints squared	(6) Col (2) × col (5)
0 –	2	0·2	0·4	0·04	0·08
0·4 –	7	0·6	4·2	0·36	2·52
0·8 –	10	1·0	10·2	1·0	10·0
1·2 –	16	1·4	22·4	1·96	31·36
1·6 –	23	1·8	41·4	3·24	74·52
2·0 –	28	2·2	61·6	4·84	135·52
2·4 –	19	2·6	49·4	6·76	128·44
2·8 –	16	3·0	48·0	9·0	144·0
3·2 –	11	3·4	37·4	11·56	127·16
3·6 –	7	3·8	26·6	14.44	101·08
4·0 –	1	4·2	4·2	17·64	17·64
4·4 –					
Total	140		305·6		772·32

As an example, Dr Green's data are set out in table 2.2, which is simply an extension of table 1.3, with two additional columns. Just as in calculating the standard deviation from ungrouped data so here we do not need to measure the actual differences between the observations and their mean. Instead we make use of the identity:

(sum of squares of differences between observations and mean) equals (sum of squares of observations) minus (sum of observations)^2 ÷ number of observations, or

$$\Sigma(x - \bar{x})^2 = \Sigma x^2 - \frac{(\Sigma x)^2}{n}$$

It is important to remember that the "observations" in this case are the midpoints in the frequency distribution.

The sum of the observations, Σx, was calculated in table 1.3 to find the mean and is now repeated in table 2.2, col (4), where the midpoint of each class of lead concentration is multiplied by the number of children in the class. Then, just as when calculating the standard deviation from the ungrouped series we squared each of the observations in turn, so now we take each of the midpoints of the observation classes shown in col (3) and square them, as in col (5). These correspond to the squares of the observations in the ungrouped series. But since we have several children in each class, shown in col (2), each squared midpoint in col (5) must be multiplied by the corresponding number of children. The result is shown in col (6), and the sum of the squares is at the foot of the column, namely, 772·32.

Continuing the procedure as for ungrouped data, we take the sum of the squares of the observations and subtract from it the sum of the observations squared divided by the number of observations. Dr Green's figures now look like this:

$$772\cdot32 - \frac{305\cdot6^2}{140}. \text{ This equals } 105\cdot239.$$

To obtain the variance we divide by $n - 1$, which is 139, and get: 0·76. The square root of that gives us the standard deviation = 0·87.

The procedure may be summarised as follows:

Set out the classes of observations in a column. Put the numbers in each class against the corresponding numbers in it. Set out the class midpoints in a column (table 2.2). Multiply the midpoint in each class by the number in the class and add them   ..   .. Σx

Square this total   ..   .. $(\Sigma x)^2$

Divide by the number of observations in all classes $\dfrac{(\Sigma x)^2}{n}$ (1)

Square each class midpoint   ..   .. x^2

Multiply each squared midpoint by the number of observations in the corresponding class and add them ..   .. Σx^2 (2)

Subtract (1) from (2) .. .. $\Sigma x^2 - \dfrac{(\Sigma x)^2}{n}$

Divide by the number of observations minus 1 .. $\dfrac{\Sigma x^2 - \dfrac{(\Sigma x)^2}{n}}{n-1}$

Take the square root .. .. $\sqrt{\dfrac{\Sigma x^2 - \dfrac{(\Sigma x)^2}{n}}{n-1}}$

This is the standard deviation.

When using a calculator it is probably best to set out at least the first three columns of table 2.2—namely, the class intervals, the numbers in each class, and the midpoints of each class. The multiplication of the midpoints by the number in each class can then proceed, the resulting products being accumulated in the memory and brought out on to the display screen when complete, to give the total at the foot of column (4).

The operations in columns (5) and (6) need not be written down. They can be carried out successively for each class, and summed in the memory to give the total at the foot of column (6). For example, in the first row of table 2.2, 0·2 is squared (=0·04 in col (5)), the square is multiplied by 2 (col (2)), and the product entered in the memory. The products derived thus from each row are accumulated in the memory, and the sum is finally obtained as 772·32, but left in the memory.

The sum of the observations is squared, 305·6², and divided by the number of observations, 140, to give 667·08. This is then subtracted from the memory and the result brought on to the display screen =105·239. This is divided by n − 1 (=139), making 0·757, and the square root taken, to give 0·87.

CONTINUOUS AND DISCRETE VARIABLES

The readings obtained of urinary concentration of lead are described as "continuous" in contrast to "discrete" or "discontinuous". This is because each reading can be any value within the possible range, the value depending on the amount of lead present and the sensitivity of the apparatus measuring it. A discrete variable is a numerical value attached to an event or finding that stands on its own and cannot take intermediate values. For example, the amount of fluid measured from a syringe can be any amount within the capacity of the syringe, and so is a continuous variable. But the number of pills taken from a bottle must be a whole number of pills, a discrete variable. Though this may seem to labour the obvious, the difference needs to be kept specially clear in the statistical treatment of data.

In tables 1.3 and 2.2 the readings are grouped in classes. Each class represents a range covering 0·4 μmol/24 h of a continuous variable. In the calculations made on the data the midpoints of each class were taken to represent the whole range of the class. But when discrete data are used, the procedure is slightly different and simpler.

For example, as well as studying the lead concentration in the urine of 140 children Dr Green asked how often each of them had been examined by a doctor at home or in his surgery during 1975. After collecting this information he tabulated the data shown in table 2.3, cols (1) and (2). He went on to calculate the mean number of visits and the standard deviation.

Clearly there can be no midpoint in the classes listed in col (1). Therefore these numbers themselves are multiplied by the numbers of children in each class to produce the figures in col (3). The total number of visits, 455, is then divided by the number of children, 140, to give the mean number of visits, 3·25.

Likewise the standard deviation would be calculated by the method shown in table 2.2 but by using the actual numbers of visits listed in 2.3, since the discrete classes have no midpoints.

For a note on "Unwieldy numbers" see Chapter 13.

TABLE 2.3—*Calculation of standard deviation from grouped data (discrete variable)*

(1) Number of visits to or from doctor	(2) Number of children	(3) Col (2) × Col (1)	(4) Col (1) squared	(5) Col (2) × Col (4)
0	2	0	0	0
1	8	8	1	8
2	27	54	4	108
3	45	135	9	405
4	38	152	16	608
5	15	75	25	375
6	4	24	36	144
7	1	7	49	49
Total	140	455		1697

Mean number of visits = $455/140 = 3\cdot25.$

Standard deviation $= \sqrt{\dfrac{1697 - \dfrac{455^2}{140}}{139}} = 1\cdot25.$

Exercise 2.1. Dr Green obtained a further series of lead concentrations in urine as follows: 0·2, 0·8, 3·1, 1·9, 0·3, 1·8, 1·7, 1·5, 3·4, 2·0, 2·1, 0·6, 1·9, 2·8, 2·0, 0·7 μmol/24 h. What is their mean and standard deviation? *Answer:* Mean = 1·675, SD = 0·96.

Exercise 2.2. In the campaign against smallpox a doctor inquired into the number of times 150 people aged 16 and over in an Ethiopian village had been vaccinated. He obtained the following figures: never, 12 people; once, 24; twice, 42; three times, 38; four times, 30; five times, 4. What is the mean number of times those people had been vaccinated and what is the standard deviation? *Answer:* Mean = 2·41, SD = 1·27.

3. Populations and samples

POPULATIONS

In statistics the term "population" has a slightly different meaning from the one given to it in ordinary speech. It need not refer only to people or to animate creatures—the population of Britain, for instance, or the dog population of London. Statisticians also speak of a population of objects, or events, or procedures, or observations, including such things as the quantity of lead in urine, visits to the doctor, or surgical operations. A population is thus an aggregate of creatures, things, cases, and so on. It also has several other properties besides this generality of meaning.

Though a statistician should clearly define the population he is dealing with, he may not be able to enumerate it exactly. For instance, in ordinary usage the population of England denotes the number of people within England's boundaries, perhaps as enumerated at a census. But a physician might embark on a study to try to answer the question, What is the average systolic blood pressure of Englishmen aged 40–59? But who are the Englishmen referred to here? Not all Englishmen live in England, and of those that do the social and genetic background may vary. Or a surgeon may study the effects of two alternative operations for gastric ulcer. But how old are the patients? What sex are they? How severe is their disease? Where do they live? And so on. The reader needs precise information on such matters if he is to draw valid inferences from the sample that was studied to the population being considered.

SAMPLES

Since a population commonly contains too many individuals to study conveniently, an investigation is often restricted to one or more samples drawn from it. A sample may therefore, like a population, consist of immaterial and abstract things as well as creatures and objects. But, to allow true inferences to be made about a population from study of a sample, the relation between the sample and the population must be such as to make that possible.

Consequently, the first important attribute of a sample is that every individual in the population from which it is drawn must have a known chance of being included in it; a natural suggestion is that these chances should be equal. To ensure this we make the choice by means of a process in which chance alone operates, such as spinning a coin or, more usually, the use of a table of random numbers. These may be consulted in several publications—for example, Armitage (1971), Hill (1971), Fisher and Yates (1974). A sample so chosen is called a *random sample*. Thus the word "random" does not describe the sample as such but the way it is selected.

To draw a satisfactory sample sometimes presents greater problems than to analyse statistically the observations made on it. A full discussion of the topic is beyond the scope of this book, but invaluable guidance is readily available in Armitage (1971) and Hill (1962, 1971). Here only an introduction is offered.

Before drawing a sample the investigator should define the population from which it is to come. Sometimes he can completely enumerate its members before he begins his analysis—for example, all the livers he has studied at necropsy over the previous year, all the patients aged 20–44 admitted to hospital with perforated peptic ulcer in the previous 20 months. In retrospective studies of this kind numbers can be allotted serially from any point in the table to each patient or specimen. Then a sample may be drawn by taking from the random numbers every even number, for instance, or every number ending in 2 or 5, and so on.

In prospective studies to be carried out on observations to be made in the future it is important to begin by defining a limit to the making of the observations. For example, a surgeon might draw one or more samples from the next 100 cases of acute appendicitis to be admitted to hospital or a general practitioner might draw one from all the cases of iron-deficiency anaemia to be seen during the next 12 months in his surgery. In studies of this kind every patient eligible for admission to the study is allotted serially a number from the table of random numbers. He is then actually admitted to the study, and perhaps assigned to one or another group within it, in accordance with a predetermined plan for using the random numbers. For example, all patients with even numbers might receive a new treatment, all patients with odd numbers receive a standard treatment.

The use of random numbers in this way is generally preferable, unless the population is very large, to taking every alternate patient or every fifth specimen or acting on some such regular plan. The regularity of the plan can occasionally coincide by chance with some unforeseen regularity in the presentation of the material for study— for example, by hospital appointments being made for patients from certain practices on certain days of the week, or specimens being prepared in batches in accordance with some schedule.

Since susceptibility to disease generally varies in relation to age, sex, occupation, family history, exposure to risk, inoculation state, country lived in or visited, and many other genetic or environmental factors, it is advisable to examine samples when drawn to see whether they are, on the average, comparable in these respects. The random process of selection is intended to make them so, but sometimes it can by chance lead to disparities between samples. To reduce the chance of some disparities the sampling may be stratified. This means that a framework is laid down initially, and the patients or objects of study in a random sample are then allotted to the compartments of the framework. For instance, the framework might have a primary division into males and females and then a secondary division of each of those categories into five age groups, the result being a framework with 10 compartments. It is then important to bear in mind that the distributions of the categories in two samples made up on such a framework may be truly comparable, but they do not reflect the distribution of these categories in the population from which the sample is drawn unless the compartments in the framework have been designed with that in mind. For instance, equal numbers might be admitted to the male and female categories, but males and females are not equally numerous in the general population, and their relative proportions in it vary with age.

VARIATION BETWEEN SAMPLES

Even if we ensure that every member of a population has a known, and usually an equal, chance of being included in a sample, it does not follow that a series of samples drawn from one population and fulfilling this criterion will be identical. They will show chance variations from one to another, and the variation may be slight or considerable. For example, a series of samples of the body temperature of healthy people would show very little variation from one to another, but the variation between samples of the systolic blood pressure would be considerable. Thus the variation between samples depends partly on the amount of variation in the population from which they are drawn.

Furthermore, it is a matter of common observation that a small sample is a much less certain guide to the population from which it was drawn than a large sample. In other words, the more members of a population that are included in a sample the more chance will that sample have of accurately representing the population, provided a random process is used to construct the sample. A consequence of this is that, if two or more samples are drawn from a population, the larger they are the more closely are they likely to resemble each other—again provided the random technique is followed. Thus the variation between samples depends partly also on the size of the sample.

3. Populations and samples 19

STANDARD ERROR OF THE MEAN

If we draw a series of samples and calculate the mean of the observations in each, we have a series of means. These means themselves generally conform to a "normal" distribution, and they often do so even if the observations from which they are obtained do not. The series of means, like the series of observations in each sample, has a standard deviation. The standard error of the mean of one sample is an estimate of the standard deviation that would be obtained from the means of a large number of samples drawn from that population.

As noted above, if a series of random samples are drawn from a population their means will vary from one to another. The variation depends on the variation in the population and the size of the sample. We do not know the variation in the population so we use as an estimate of it the variation in the sample. This is expressed in the standard deviation. If we now divide the standard deviation by the square root of the number of observations in the sample we have an estimate of the standard error of the mean. $SEM = SD/\sqrt{n}$.

Dr Louise White is a general practitioner in Yorkshire. Her practice includes part of a town with a large printing works and some of the adjacent sheep farming country. With her patients' informed consent she has been investigating whether the diastolic blood pressure of men aged 20 to 44 differs between the printers and the farm workers. For this purpose she has obtained a random sample of 72 printers and 48 farm workers and calculated the means and standard deviations as shown in table 3.1.

TABLE 3.1—*Mean diastolic blood pressures in mm Hg of printers and farmers*

	Number	Mean diastolic blood pressure	Standard deviation
Printers	72	88	4·5
Farmers	48	79	4·2

To calculate the standard errors of the two mean blood pressures the standard deviation of each sample is divided by the square root of the number of the observations in the sample.

Printers: $SEM = 4·5/\sqrt{72} = 0·53$ mm Hg.

Farmers: $SEM = 4·2/\sqrt{48} = 0·61$ mm Hg.

These standard errors may be used to study the significance of the difference between the two means, as described below (p 25).

NOT A RANDOM SAMPLE

It is now convenient to consider another problem arising from Dr Green's studies. His sample of 15 children had a mean urinary lead concentration of 1·5 μmol/24 h. Can he generalise from this and say anything valid about the whole 140 children's urinary lead concentration? The answer is No. The 15 children were all the children in one street. Children living in other streets of the housing estate had no chance of inclusion in the sample, so it is not a random sample of those 140 children. The mean of 1·5 μmol/24 h found for the 15 children therefore does not indicate what the mean of the whole population of 140 children may be. The population mean was in fact 2·18, and the sample mean in this case cannot be validly compared with it. Moreover, the 15 children were included in the 140, so if their mean urinary lead concentration is included in the mean for the 140, the observations derived from the 15 are counted twice. This also complicates any comparison Dr Green might try to make between the two sets of data.

Exercise 3. Dr Green found that the mean urinary lead concentration in 140 children was 2·18 μmol/24 h, with standard deviation 0·87. What is the standard error of the mean? *Answer:* 0·074

4. Statements of probability

We have seen that when a set of observations have a "normal" distribution multiples of the standard deviation mark certain limits on the scatter of the observations. For instance, 1·96 (or approximately 2) standard deviations above and 1·96 standard deviations below the mean ($\bar{x} \pm 1\cdot96$ SD) mark the points within which 95% of the observations lie.

We noted that Dr Green's 140 children had a mean urinary lead concentration of 2·18 μmol/24 h, with standard deviation 0·87. The 95% probability limits here are 2·18 $\pm$ (1·96 × 0·87), giving a range of 0·47 to 3·89. One of the children had a urinary lead concentration of just over 4·0 μmol/24 h. This observation is greater than 3·89 and so falls in the 5% beyond the 95% probability limits. We can say that the probability of each of such observations occurring is 5% or less. This probability is usually expressed as a fraction of 1 rather than of 100, and written P < 0·05.

Standard deviations (or standard errors, which behave in exactly the same way) thus set limits about which probability statements can be made. Some of these are set out in table A (Appendix). To use table A to estimate the probability of finding an observed value, say a urinary lead concentration of 4·8 μmol/24 h, in sampling from the same population of observations as Dr Green's 140 children provided, we proceed as follows.

The mean of Dr Green's series was 2·18 μmol/24 h, and the standard deviation 0·87. How many standard deviations from the mean does the new observation lie? The distance of the new observation from the mean is 4·8 − 2·18 = 2·62. How many standard deviations does this represent? Dividing the difference by the standard deviation gives 2·62/0·87 = 3·01. This number is greater than 2·576 in the table but less than 3·291, so the probability of finding a deviation as large as this lies between 0·01 and 0·001, which may be expressed as 0·01 > P > 0·001. In fact table A shows that the probability is very close to 0·0027. This probability is small, so the observation probably did not come from the same population.

Again, the mean number of times that Dr Green's 140 children saw a doctor in one year (table 2.3) was 3·25, with a standard deviation of 1·25. A child that Dr Green thought needed special study was seen by a doctor only once. Was this unusual? The difference between this one visit and the mean is $3·25 - 1 = 2·25$. How many standard deviations does this represent? $2·25/1·25 = 1·8$. Table A shows that 1·8 standard deviations correspond to a probability of between 0·1 and 0·05. This is more than 5%, and so fairly high. Therefore this child's one visit was not particularly unusual in relation to the numbers of visits to or from their doctors that the 140 children had as a whole.

To take another example, Dr White found the mean diastolic blood pressure of the printers to be 88 mm Hg and the standard deviation 4·5 mm Hg. One of the printers had a diastolic blood pressure of 100 mm Hg. The mean plus or minus 1·96 times its standard deviation gives the following two figures:

$$88 + (1·96 \times 4·5) = 96·8 \text{ mm Hg}$$
$$88 - (1·96 \times 4·5) = 79·2 \text{ mm Hg}.$$

We can say therefore that only 1 in 20 (or 5%) of printers in the population from which the sample is drawn would be expected to have a diastolic blood pressure below about 79 or above about 97 mm Hg. These are the 95% limits. The 99·73% limits lie 3 standard deviations below and 3 above the mean. The blood pressure of 100 mm Hg noted in one printer thus lies beyond the 95% limit of 97 but within the 99·73% limit of 101·5 ($= 88 + (3 \times 4·5)$). This sort of difference from the mean is commonly described as "significant". That is to say, it is significant at the 5% level because the observation lies beyond the 95% limit set by 1·96 standard deviations.

The means and their standard errors can be treated similarly. If a series of samples are drawn and the mean of each calculated, 95% of the means would be expected to fall within the range of two standard errors above and two below the mean of these means. This common mean would be expected to lie very close to the mean of the population. So the standard error of a mean provides a statement of probability about the difference between the mean of the population and the mean of the sample.

CONFIDENCE LIMITS

Confidence limits provide the key to a useful device for arguing from a sample back to the population from which it came. For example, Dr White found in her sample of 72 printers a mean diastolic blood pressure of 88 mm Hg. The standard error of the mean was 0·53

4. Statements of probability 23

mm Hg. The sample mean plus or minus 1·96 times its standard error gives the following two figures:

$$88 + (1·96 \times 0·53) = 89·04 \text{ mm Hg}$$
$$88 - (1·96 \times 0·53) = 86·96 \text{ mm Hg.}$$

These are called 95% *confidence limits*, and we can say that there is only a 5% chance that the range of 86·96 to 89·04 mm Hg excludes the mean of the population. Then if we take the mean plus or minus three times its standard error, the range would be from 86·41 to 89·59. These are the 99·73% confidence limits, and the chance of this range excluding the population mean is 1 in 370.

With small samples—say, under 30 observations—somewhat larger multiples of the standard error are needed to set confidence limits. This subject is discussed below under the t distribution (Chapter 7).

Exercise 4.1. A count of malaria parasites in 100 fields with a 2-mm oil immersion lens gave a mean of 35 parasites per field, standard deviation 11·6 (the counts are assumed to follow a normal distribution). On counting one more field the pathologist found 52 parasites. Does this number lie outside the 95% probability limits; what are they? *Answer:* No; 12·26 and 57·74.

Exercise 4.2. What are the 95% confidence limits for the mean of the population from which this sample count of parasites was drawn? *Answer:* 32·73 and 37·27.

5. Differences between means

We saw in Chapter 3 that the mean of a sample has a standard error, and a mean that departs by more than twice its standard error from the population mean would be expected by chance only in about 5% of samples. Likewise the difference between the means of two samples also has a standard error. We do not normally know the population mean, so we may suppose that the mean of one of our samples estimates it. The sample mean may happen to be identical with the population mean. More likely it lies somewhere above or below the population mean, and there is a 95% chance that it is within 1·96 standard errors above or below it.

Consider now the mean of the second sample. If the sample comes from the same population its mean will also have a 95% chance of lying within 1·96 standard errors above or below the population mean. But if we do not know the population mean we have only the means of our samples to guide us. Therefore, if we want to know whether they are likely to have come from the same population, we ask, Do they lie within a certain range, represented by their standard errors, of each other?

STANDARD ERROR OF DIFFERENCE BETWEEN MEANS

If SD_1 represents the standard deviation of sample 1 and SD_2 the standard deviation of sample 2, and n_1 the number in sample 1 and n_2 the number in sample 2, the formula denoting the standard error of the difference between two means is:

$$SE\ diff = \sqrt{\frac{SD_1^2}{n_1} + \frac{SD_2^2}{n_2}}$$

The computation is straightforward.

Square the standard deviation of sample 1 and divide by the number of observations in the sample   .. $\dfrac{SD_1^2}{n_1}$ (1)

Square the standard deviation of sample 2 and divide by the number of observations in the sample   .. $\dfrac{SD_2^2}{n_2}$ (2)

Add (1) and (2)   ..   .. $\dfrac{SD_1^2}{n_1} + \dfrac{SD_2^2}{n_2}$

Take the square root .. .. $\sqrt{\dfrac{SD_1{}^2}{n_1} + \dfrac{SD_2{}^2}{n_2}}$

This is the standard error of the difference between the two means.

An example of its calculation with Dr White's figures is given below, but first a note on the so-called null hypothesis is needed.

NULL HYPOTHESIS

In comparing the mean blood pressures of the printers and the farmers we are testing the hypothesis that the two samples came from the same population of blood pressures. The hypothesis that there is no difference between the population from which the printers' blood pressures were drawn and the population from which the farmers' blood pressures were drawn is called the null hypothesis.

But what do we mean by "no difference"? Chance alone will almost certainly ensure that there is some difference between the *sample* means, for they are most unlikely to be identical. Consequently we set limits within which we shall regard the samples as not having any significant difference. If we set the limits at twice the standard error of the difference, and regard a mean outside this range as coming from another population, we shall on average be wrong about once in 20 times if the null hypothesis is in fact true. For we know that, when data are normally distributed, about 5% in a single population will by chance alone be outside the range of two standard deviations from the mean. Likewise if we allow a difference of three times the standard error of the difference, and regard a mean outside this range as coming from another population, we shall on average be wrong once in 370 times.

A range of not more than two standard errors is often taken as implying "no difference". But there is nothing to stop an investigator choosing a range of three standard errors (or more) if he wants to reduce his chances of rejecting the null hypothesis on the basis of an aberrant observation.

A point to note here is that we try to show that a null hypothesis is *unlikely*, not its converse, that it is likely. So a difference which is greater than the limits we have set, and which we therefore regard as "significant", makes the null hypothesis *unlikely*. A difference within the limits we have set, and which we therefore regard as "non-significant", does not make the hypothesis likely.

COMPARISON OF TWO MEANS

Dr White wants to compare the mean of the printers' blood pressures with the mean of the farmers' blood pressures. Therefore she erects

c

the null hypothesis that there is no significant difference between them. The figures are set out first as in table 5.1 (which repeats table 3.1).

TABLE 5.1—*Mean diastolic blood pressures in mm Hg of printers and farmers*

	Number	Mean diastolic blood pressure	Standard deviation
Printers	72	88	4·5
Farmers	48	79	4·2

Analysing these figures in accordance with the formula given above, we have:

$$\text{SE diff} = \sqrt{\frac{4\cdot5^2}{72} + \frac{4\cdot2^2}{48}} = 0\cdot81 \text{ mm Hg.}$$

The difference between the means is $88 - 79 = 9$ mm Hg. We now find how many multiples of its standard error this difference represents: $9 \div 0\cdot81 = 11\cdot1$. Reference to table A shows that this is far beyond the figure of 3·291 standard deviations representing a probability of 0·001 (or 1 in a thousand). The probability of a difference of 11·1 standard errors occurring by chance is therefore exceedingly low, and correspondingly the null hypothesis that these two samples came from the same population of observations is exceedingly unlikely. The probability may be written $P \ll 0\cdot001$.

Sometimes a mean may be known from a very large number of observations and the investigator wants to compare the mean of his sample with it. We may not know the standard deviation of the large number of observations or the standard error of their mean. But this need not hinder the comparison if we can assume that the standard error of the mean of the large number of observations is near 0 or at least very small in relation to the standard error of the mean of the small sample.

This is because the formula for calculating the standard error of the difference between the two means—

$\sqrt{\dfrac{SD_1{}^2}{n_1} + \dfrac{SD_2{}^2}{n_2}}$ has n_1 so large that $\dfrac{SD_1{}^2}{n_1}$ becomes so small as to be neg-

ligible. The formula thus reduces to $\sqrt{\dfrac{SD_2{}^2}{n_2}}$, which is the same as that

for the standard error of the mean (p 19), namely $\dfrac{SD_2}{\sqrt{n_2}}$.

Consequently we find the standard error of the mean of the sample and divide it into the difference between the means.

For example, a large number of observations has shown that the mean count of erythrocytes in men is $5.5 \times 10^{12}/l$. In a sample of 100 men a mean count of 5.35 was found with standard deviation 1.1. The standard error of this mean is $SD/\sqrt{n}$, so that $1.1/\sqrt{100} = 0.11$. The difference between the two means is $5.5 - 5.35 = 0.15$. This difference divided by the standard error is $0.15/0.11 = 1.36$. This figure is well below the 5% level of 1.96 and in fact is below the 10% level of 1.645 (see table A). Consequently we conclude that the difference is of no statistical significance.

Exercise 5.1. In one group of 62 patients with iron-deficiency anaemia the haemoglobin level was 12.2 g/dl, standard deviation 1.8 g/dl; and in another group of 35 patients it was 10.9 g/dl, standard deviation 2.1 g/dl. What is the standard error of the difference, and what is the significance of the difference? *Answer:* 0.42 g/dl, $0.01 > P > 0.001$.

Exercise 5.2. If the mean haemoglobin level in the general population is taken as 14.4 g/dl, what is the standard error of the difference between the mean of the first sample and the population mean and what is the significance of the difference? *Answer:* 0.23 g/dl, $P < 0.001$.

6. Percentages and paired alternatives

STANDARD ERROR OF A PERCENTAGE

Just as a mean and a difference between two means can have standard errors so can a percentage and a difference between two percentages. Again both the size of the sample and the amount of variation in the population from which it is drawn affect the size of the standard error.

For example, Mr Black is a senior surgical registrar in a large hospital in Edinburgh. He is investigating acute appendicitis in people aged 65 and over. As a preliminary study he examines the hospital case notes over the previous ten years and finds that of 120 patients in this age group, with a diagnosis confirmed at operation, 73 were women and 47 were men. The percentages are: women 60·8%, men 39·2%.

If p represents one percentage, 100 − p represents the other. Then the standard error of each of these percentages is obtained by (1) multiplying them together, (2) dividing the product by the number in the sample, and (3) taking the square root:

$$\text{SE percentage} = \sqrt{\frac{p(100 - p)}{n}}.$$

Mr Black's figures are as follows:

$$\text{SE percentage} = \sqrt{\frac{60·8 \times 39·2}{120}} = 4·46.$$

With this standard error we can get 95% confidence limits on the two percentages:

60·8 ± (1·96 × 4·46) = 52·1 and 69·5

39·2 ± (1·96 × 4·46) = 30·5 and 47·9.

There is a probability of 95% that the percentages of men and women in the population from which the sample came fall within these confidence limits.

STANDARD ERROR OF DIFFERENCE BETWEEN PERCENTAGES

Mr Black wonders whether the percentages of men and women in his sample differ from the percentages of all the other men and women aged 65 and over admitted to the surgical wards during the same period. After excluding his sample of appendicitis cases, so that they are not counted twice, he makes a rough estimate of the number of patients admitted in those 10 years and finds it to be about 12000 to 13000. He therefore selects every twentieth case and so obtains a sample of 640 patients. Of these, 363 were women and 277 men, giving percentages of 56·7 for women and 43·3 for men.

The percentage of women in the appendicitis sample differs from the percentage of women in the general surgical sample by 60·8 — 56·7 = 4·1%. Is this difference of any significance?

There are two ways of calculating the standard error of the difference between two percentages. One is theoretically more soundly based for the problem we are considering—testing a null hypothesis. The other is in practice more readily calculated and usually gives almost the same result.

The following formula gives the theoretically preferable method:

$$\text{SE diff }\% = \sqrt{\frac{p \times (100 - p)}{n_1} + \frac{p \times (100 - p)}{n_2}}.$$

To obtain p we must amalgamate the two samples and calculate the percentage of women in the two combined; $100 - p$ is then the percentage of men in the two combined. n_1 and n_2 are the numbers in each sample.

Number of women in the samples: $73 + 363 = 436$

Number of people in the samples: $120 + 640 = 760$

% of women: $(436 \times 100)/760 = 57·4$

% of men: $(324 \times 100)/760 = 42·6$

Putting these numbers in the formula, we find the standard error of the difference between the percentages is

$$\sqrt{\frac{57·4 \times 42·6}{120} + \frac{57·4 \times 42·6}{640}} = 4·92.$$

In practice it is generally simpler to use the percentages in each sample as in the following formula:

$$\sqrt{\frac{p_1 \times (100 - p_1)}{n_1} + \frac{p_2 \times (100 - p_2)}{n_2}}.$$

With Mr Black's figures we have:

$$\sqrt{\frac{60·8 \times 39·2}{120} + \frac{56·7 \times 43·3}{640}} = 4·87.$$

The results obtained by these two methods differ in this case by only 0·05, which is negligible.

The difference between the percentage of women (and men) in the two samples was 4·1%. To find the probability attached to this difference we divide it by its standard error (obtained by the first, more accurate method above): $4\cdot1/4\cdot92 = 0\cdot83$. As this ratio is less than one standard error, the difference between the percentages in the two samples could have been due to chance alone.

STANDARD ERROR OF A TOTAL

The total number of deaths from a particular disease varies from year to year in a town. When the population of the town or the area where they occur is fairly large, say, some thousands, and provided the deaths are independent of one another, the standard error of the number of deaths from a specified cause is given approximately by its square root, $\sqrt{n}$. Further, the standard error of the difference between two numbers of deaths, n_1 and n_2, can be taken as $\sqrt{n_1 + n_2}$. This can be used to estimate the significance of a difference between two

totals by dividing the difference by its standard error: $\dfrac{n_1 - n_2}{\sqrt{n_1 + n_2}}$.

It is important to note that the deaths themselves must be independently caused; for example, they must not be the result of an epidemic such as influenza. And the reports of the deaths must likewise be independent; for example, the criteria for diagnosis must be consistent from year to year and not suddenly changed in accordance with a new fashion or test.

Despite its limitations this method has its uses. For instance, in Carlisle the number of deaths from ischaemic heart disease in 1973 was 276. Is this significantly higher than the total for 1972, which was 246? The difference is 30. The standard error of the difference is $\sqrt{276 + 246} = 22\cdot8$. We then take $30 \div 22\cdot8 = 1\cdot313$. This is clearly much less than $1\cdot96$ times the standard error at the 5% level of probability. Reference to table A shows that in fact $P > 0\cdot1$. The difference could therefore easily be a chance fluctuation.

This method should be regarded as giving no more than approximate but useful guidance, and is unlikely to be valid over a period of more than very few years owing to changes in diagnostic techniques. An extension of it to the study of paired alternatives follows.

PAIRED ALTERNATIVES

Sometimes it is possible to record the results of treatment or some sort of test or investigation as one of two alternatives. For instance, two treatments or tests might be carried out on pairs obtained by matching individuals chosen by random sampling. Or the pairs might consist of successive treatments of the same individual (see p 38 for comparison of pairs by the *t* test). The results might then be recorded as " responded or did not respond", "improved or did not improve", "positive or negative", and so on.

This type of study yields results that can be set out as follows:

Member of pair receiving treatment A	Member of pair receiving treatment B
Responded	Responded (1)
Responded	Did not respond (2)
Did not respond	Responded (3)
Did not respond	Did not respond (4)

The significance of the results can then be simply tested by McNemar's test in the following way.

Ignore rows (1) and (4), and examine rows (2) and (3). Let the larger number of pairs in either of rows (2) or (3) be called n_1 and the smaller number of pairs in either of those two rows be n_2. We may then calculate

$\frac{n_1 - n_2}{\sqrt{n_1 + n_2}}$. The result is normally distributed, and its probability can be read from table A.

However, in practice, the fairly small numbers that form the subject of this type of investigation make a correction advisable. We therefore diminish the difference between n_1 and n_2 by 1, using the following

formula: $\frac{(n_1 - n_2) - 1}{\sqrt{n_1 + n_2}}$.

Again, the result is normally distributed, and its probability can be read from table A.

For example, Dr Katherine Grey is a registrar in the gastro-enterological unit of a large hospital in an industrial city. She sees a considerable number of patients with severe recurrent aphthous ulcer of the mouth. Claims have been made that a recently introduced pre-paration stops the pain of these ulcers and promotes quicker healing than existing preparations.

Over a period of six months she therefore selected every patient with this disorder and paired them off so far as possible by reference to age, sex, and frequency of ulceration. Finally she had 108 patients in 54 pairs. To one member of each pair she gave treatment A, which she and her colleagues in the unit had hitherto regarded as the best; to the other member she gave the new treatment, B. Both forms of treatment are local applications, and they cannot be made to look alike. Con-sequently to avoid bias in the assessment of the results a colleague

recorded the results of treatment without knowing which patient in
each pair had which treatment. The results are shown in table 6.1.

TABLE 6.1—*Results of treating aphthous ulcer in 54 pairs of patients*

Member of pair receiving treatment A	Member of pair receiving treatment B	Pairs of patients
Responded	Responded	16
Responded	Did not respond	23
Did not respond	Responded	10
Did not respond	Did not respond	5
	Total	54

Here $n_1 = 23$, $n_2 = 10$. Entering these values in the formula given
above we have $\dfrac{(23 - 10) - 1}{\sqrt{23 + 10}} = \dfrac{12}{\sqrt{33}} = 2\cdot089$.

The 5% level of probability is at 1·96 standard deviations (table A).
Here 2·089 exceeds that. Therefore we may conclude that treatment A,
the traditional treatment, gave significantly better results than treatment
B, the new one.

Exercise 6.1. In an obstetric hospital 17·8% of 320 women were delivered
by forceps in 1975. What is the standard error of this percentage? *Answer:*
2·1%. In another hospital in the same region 21·2% of 185 women were
delivered by forceps. What is the standard error of the difference between the
percentages at this hospital and the first? *Answer:* 3·7% What is the difference
between these percentages of forceps delivery and what is its significance?
Answer: 3·4%; 0·5 > P > 0·3.

Exercise 6.2. A dermatologist tested a new topical application for the treatment
of psoriasis on 47 patients. He applied it to the lesions on one part of the
patient's body and what he considered to be the best traditional remedy to the
lesions on another but comparable part of the body. In three patients both
areas of psoriasis responded; in 28 patients the disease responded to the traditional remedy but hardly or not at all to the new one; in 13 it responded to the
new one but hardly or not at all to the traditional remedy; and in four cases
neither remedy caused an appreciable response. Did either remedy cause a
significantly better response than the other? *Answer:* Yes, the traditional
remedy; 0·05 > P > 0·01.

7. The t tests

Previously we have considered how to test the null hypotheses that there is no difference between the mean of a sample and the population mean, and no difference between the means of two samples. We obtained the difference between the means by subtraction, and then divided this difference by the standard error of the difference. If the difference is 1·96 times its standard error, or more, it is likely to occur with a frequency of only 1 in 20, or less. The probability attached to other ratios of the difference divided by the standard error appears in table A.

But with small samples, where more chance variation must be allowed for, these ratios are not entirely accurate. Some modification of the procedure of dividing the difference by its standard error is needed, and the technique to use is the t test. Its foundations were laid by W S Gosset under the pseudonym "Student" (1908) so that it is sometimes known as Student's t test. The procedure does not differ greatly from the one used for large samples, but it is preferable when the number of observations is fewer than about 60, and certainly when they amount to only 30 or less.

The application of the t distribution to four types of problem will now be considered:

(1) The mean and standard deviation of a sample are known (or can be calculated). What is the probability that a certain range round the sample mean includes the population mean?

(2) The mean and standard deviation of a sample are known (or can be calculated) and a value is postulated for the mean of the population. How significantly does the sample mean differ from the postulated population mean?

(3) The means and standard deviations of two samples are known (or can be calculated). How significant is the difference between the means?

(4) Paired observations are made on two samples (or in succession on one sample). What is the significance of the difference between the means of the two sets of observations?

In each case the problem is essentially the same—namely, to establish multiples of standard errors to which probabilities can be attached. These multiples are the number of times a difference can be divided by its standard error. We have seen that with large samples 1·96 times the standard error has a probability of 5% or less, and 2·576 times the standard error a probability of 1% or less (table A). With small samples these multiples of standard error are larger, and the smaller the sample the larger they become.

(1) WHERE DOES POPULATION MEAN LIE?

A rare congenital disease, Everley's syndrome, generally causes a reduction in concentration of blood sodium. This is thought to provide a useful diagnostic sign as well as a clue to the efficacy of treatment. Little is known about the subject, but Dr Pink, who is director of a dermatological department in a London teaching hospital, is known to be interested in the disease and has seen more cases than anyone else. Even so, he has seen only 18. The patients were all aged between 20 and 44.

From study of his 18 cases Dr Pink has found that their mean blood sodium concentration was 155 mmol/l, with standard deviation of 12 mmol/l. For future guidance where may one expect the mean to lie in cases of this disease? What are the 95% confidence limits within which the mean of the total population of such cases may be expected to lie?

Dr Pink's data are set out as follows:

Number of observations   18

Mean blood sodium concentration . .   . .   . . 115 mmol/l

Standard deviation   . .   . .   12 mmol/l

Standard error of mean $SD/\sqrt{n} = 12/\sqrt{18} =$ 2·83 mmol/l

To find the 95% confidence limits above and below the mean we now have to find a multiple of the standard error. In large samples we have seen that the multiple is 1·96 (Chapter 4). For small samples we use the table of t. As the sample becomes smaller t becomes larger for any particular level of probability. Conversely, as the sample becomes larger t becomes smaller and approaches the values given in table A, reaching them for infinitely large samples.

Since the size of the sample influences t it is taken into account in relating it to probabilities in the table. Some useful parts of the full t table appear in table B (Appendix). The left-hand column is headed DF for "degrees of freedom". The use of these was noted in the calculation of the standard deviation (Chapter 2). In practice they amount in these circumstances to 1 less than the number of observations in the sample. With Dr Pink's data we have $18 - 1 = 17$. This is because only 17 observations plus the total number of observations are needed to specify the sample, the 18th being determined by subtraction.

To find the number by which we must multiply the standard error to give the 95% confidence limits we enter the table at 17 in the left-hand column and read across to the column headed 0·05. There the number 2·110 appears. The 95% confidence limits of the mean are now set as follows:

Mean + 2·110 SE
Mean − 2·110 SE.

Dr Pink's figures come out as follows:

$115 + (2{\cdot}110 \times 2{\cdot}83) = 120{\cdot}97$ mmol/l
$115 - (2{\cdot}110 \times 2{\cdot}83) = 109{\cdot}03$ mmol/l.

We may then say, with a 95% chance of being correct, that the range 109·03 to 120·97 mmol/l includes the population mean.

Likewise from table B the 1% confidence limits of the mean are as follows:

Mean + 2·898 SE
Mean − 2·898 SE.

Dr Pink's figures have the following limits at the 1% probability level:

$115 + (2{\cdot}898 \times 2{\cdot}83) = 123{\cdot}20$
$115 - (2{\cdot}898 \times 2{\cdot}83) = 106{\cdot}80$.

(2) DIFFERENCE OF SAMPLE MEAN FROM POPULATION MEAN

Estimations of plasma calcium concentration in Dr Pink's 18 patients with Everley's syndrome gave a mean of 3·2 mmol/l, with standard deviation 1·1. Previous experience from a number of investigations and published reports had shown that the mean was commonly close to 2.5 mmol/l in healthy people aged 20–44, the age range of Dr Pink's patients. Is the mean in his patients abnormally high?

We set the figures out as follows:

Mean of general population, μ	2·5 mmol/l
Mean of sample, $\bar{x}$	3·2 mmol/l
Standard deviation of sample, SD	1·1 mmol/l
Standard error of sample mean, $\text{SD}/\sqrt{n} = 1{\cdot}1\sqrt{18}$	0·26 mmol/l
Difference between means, $\mu - \bar{x} = 2{\cdot}5 - 3{\cdot}2$ ..	− 0·7 mmol/l

t = difference between means divided by standard

error of sample mean $\dfrac{\mu - \bar{x}}{\text{SD}/\sqrt{n}} = \dfrac{-\,0{\cdot}7}{0{\cdot}26} = -\,2{\cdot}69$

Degrees of freedom, $n - 1 = 18 - 1 = 17$.

Ignoring the sign of the *t* value, and entering table B at 17 degrees of freedom, we find that 2·69 comes between probability values of 0·02 and 0·01, in other words between 2% and 1%. It is therefore unlikely that the sample with mean 3·2 came from the population with mean 2·5, and we may conclude that the sample mean is, at least statistically, unusually high. Whether it should be regarded clinically as abnormally high is something that needs to be considered separately by the physician in charge of that case.

(3) DIFFERENCE BETWEEN MEANS OF TWO SAMPLES

Here we apply a modified procedure for finding the standard error of the difference between two means and testing the size of the difference by this standard error (see Chapter 5 for large samples). For large samples we used the standard deviation of each sample, computed separately, to calculate the standard error of the difference between the means. For small samples we calculate a combined standard deviation for the two samples. The following example illustrates the procedure.

The addition of bran to the diet has been reported to benefit patients with diverticulosis. Several different bran preparations are available, and Dr Silver wants to test the efficacy of two of them on his patients, since favourable claims have been made for each. Among the consequences of administering bran that he wants to test is the transit time

TABLE 7.1—*Transit times in hours of marker pellets through alimentary canal of patients with diverticulosis on two types of treatment: unpaired comparison*

	Transit times in hours	
	Sample 1 Treatment A	Sample 2 Treatment B
	44	52
	51	64
	52	68
	55	74
	60	79
	62	83
	66	84
	68	88
	69	95
	71	97
	71	101
	76	116
	82	
	91	
	108	
Total	1026	1001
Mean	68·40	83·42

through the alimentary canal. Does it differ in the two groups of patients taking these two preparations of bran?

Dr Silver assumes the null hypothesis that there is no difference. By a random method he selects two groups of patients aged 40 to 64 with diverticulosis of comparable severity. Sample 1 contains 15 patients who are given treatment A, and sample 2 contains 12 patients who are given treatment B. The transit times of food through the gut are measured by a standard technique with marked pellets and the results are recorded, in order of increasing time, in table 7.1.

With treatment A the mean transit time was 68·40 h and with treatment B 83·42 h. What is the significance of the difference, 15·02 h? The procedure is as follows:

Find the sum of the squares of the observations in sample 1 Σx_1^2
Find the sum of the squares of the observations in sample 2 Σx_2^2
Find the square of the total of the observations in sample 1 $(\Sigma x_1)^2$
Find the square of the total of the observations in sample 2 $(\Sigma x_2)^2$
Divide the square of the total of the observations in sample 1
   by the number in sample 1   ..   ..   .. $\dfrac{(\Sigma x_1)^2}{n_1}$

Divide the square of the total of the observations in sample 2
   by the number in sample 2   ..   ..   .. $\dfrac{(\Sigma x_2)^2}{n_2}$

For each sample find the sum of the squares of the difference from their respective means:

$$\Sigma(x_1 - \bar{x}_1)^2 = \Sigma x_1^2 - \frac{(\Sigma x_1)^2}{n_1}; \ \Sigma(x_2 - \bar{x}_2)^2 = \Sigma x_2^2 - \frac{(\Sigma x_2)^2}{n_2}.$$

The square of the standard deviation (variance) for the two samples combined is now as follows:

$$\frac{\Sigma(x_1 - \bar{x}_1)^2 + \Sigma(x_2 - \bar{x}_2)^2}{(n_1 - 1) + (n_2 - 1)} = SD^2.$$

The divisors $n_1 - 1$ and $n_2 - 1$ represent degrees of freedom. They are referred to briefly above and in these circumstances are 1 less than the total in the sample.

The standard error of the difference between the means is

$$SE\ diff = \sqrt{\frac{SD^2}{n_1} + \frac{SD^2}{n_2}}$$

When the difference between the means is divided by this standard error the result is *t*.

$$\text{Thus } t = \frac{\bar{x}_1 - \bar{x}_2}{\sqrt{\dfrac{SD^2}{n_1} + \dfrac{SD^2}{n_4}}}.$$

The table of the t distribution (table B) is entered at $(n_1 - 1) + (n_2 - 1)$ degrees of freedom.

Dr Silver's figures work out like this:

		Treatment A	Treatment B
n	$=$	15	12
Σx	$=$	1026	1001
$\bar{x}$	$=$	68·4	83·42
Σx^2	$=$	73978	86921
$(\Sigma x)^2$	$=$	1052676	1002001
$\dfrac{(\Sigma x)^2}{n}$	$=$	70178·4	83500·083
$\Sigma(x - \bar{x})^2 =$		3799·6	3420·917

$$SD^2 = \frac{3799·6 + 3420·917}{(15 - 1) + (12 - 1)} = 288·82$$

$$SE\ diff = \sqrt{\frac{288·82}{15} + \frac{288·82}{12}}$$

$$= \sqrt{288·82\left(\frac{1}{15} + \frac{1}{12}\right)}$$

$$= 6·582$$

$$t = \frac{83·42 - 68·4}{6·582} = 2·282$$

The table of t distribution shows that at 25 degrees of freedom, that is $(15 - 1) + (12 - 1)$, when $t = 2·282$, it lies between 2·060 and 2·485. Consequently, $0·05 > P > 0·02$.

This degree of probability is just smaller than the conventional level of 5%. The null hypothesis that there is no significant difference between the means is therefore somewhat unlikely.

(4) DIFFERENCE BETWEEN MEANS OF PAIRED SAMPLES

When comparing the effects of two alternative treatments or experiments it is sometimes possible to make comparisons in pairs. For example, we may want to compare a new treatment with a traditional treatment or a new test with a standard one. Two courses are possible. Firstly, we may use the same sample twice over, so that each member of it receives both treatments, acting as his own control. Secondly, we may draw two samples and, before any treatment is started, pair each member of one with a member of the other, giving treatment A to all the members of sample 1 and treatment B to their pairs in sample 2.

The first case to consider is when each member of the sample acts as his own control. Whether treatment A or treatment B is given first or second to each member of the sample should be determined by the use of a table of random numbers. In this way any effect of one treatment on the other, even indirectly through the patient's attitude to treatment, for instance, can be minimised. Occasionally it is possible to give both treatments simultaneously, as in the treatment of a skin disease by applying a remedy to the skin on opposite sides of the body.

For example, Dr Silver is continuing his studies of bran in the treatment of diverticulosis. Having chosen the preparation that he found induced the shorter alimentary transit time, he wonders whether this transit time would be even shorter if the bran is given in the same dosage in three meals during the day (treatment A) or in one meal (treatment B). He chooses a random sample of patients with disease of comparable severity and aged 20–44, and administers the two treatments to them on two successive occasions, the order of the treatments also being determined from the table of random numbers. The alimentary transit times and the differences for each pair of treatments are set out in table 7.2.

TABLE 7.2—*Transit times in hours of marker pellets through alimentary canal of 12 patients with diverticulosis on two types of treatment: paired comparison*

| Patient | Transit times in hours | | Difference A–B |
	Treatment A	Treatment B	
1	63	55	8
2	54	62	— 8
3	79	108	— 29
4	68	77	— 9
5	87	83	4
6	84	78	6
7	92	79	13
8	57	94	— 37
9	66	69	— 3
10	53	66	— 13
11	76	72	4
12	63	77	— 14
Total	842	920	— 78
Mean	70·17	76·67	— 6·5

In calculating t on the paired observations we work with the difference, d, between the members of each pair. Our first task is to find the mean of the differences between the observations and then the standard error of the mean, proceeding as follows:

Find the sum of the differences ... Σd

Find the mean of the differences ... $\bar{d}$

Find the sum of the squares of the differences ... ... Σd^2 (1)

Find the square of the sum of the differences ... ... $(\Sigma d)^2$

Divide the square of the sum of the differences by the number (n) of differences ... ... $\dfrac{(\Sigma d)^2}{n}$ (2)

Subtract (2) from (1) ... ... $\Sigma d^2 - \dfrac{(\Sigma d)^2}{n} = \Sigma(d - \bar{d})^2$

Divide by the number of degrees of freedom (n − 1) ... ... $\dfrac{\Sigma d^2 - \dfrac{(\Sigma d)^2}{n}}{n - 1}$

This gives the square of the standard deviation (variance) ... ... SD^2

Divide the variance by the number of differences ... ... $\dfrac{SD^2}{n}$

Take the square root ... ... $\sqrt{\dfrac{SD^2}{n}}$

This is the standard error of the mean of the differences.

To calculate t, divide the mean of the differences by the standard error of the mean:

$$t = \bar{d} \div \sqrt{\dfrac{SD^2}{n}}.$$

The table of the t distribution is entered at n − 1 degrees of freedom (number of pairs minus 1).

Dr Silver's figures are treated as follows:

n	12
Σd	− 78
$\bar{d}$	− 6·5
Σd^2	3030
$\dfrac{(\Sigma d)^2}{n}$	507
$\Sigma d^2 - \dfrac{(\Sigma d)^2}{n}$	2523

Divide by n — 1 to give SD^2 ..   ..   229·36

SE mean difference $= \sqrt{\dfrac{\text{SD}^2}{\text{n}}} = \sqrt{\dfrac{229 \cdot 36}{12}} = 4 \cdot 37$

$t = -6 \cdot 5 \div 4 \cdot 37 = -1 \cdot 487.$

Entering the table of the *t* distribution at 11 degrees of freedom (that is, n — 1) and ignoring the minus sign, we find that this value lies between 0·697 and 1·796. Reading off the probability value, we see that $0 \cdot 5 > P > 0 \cdot 1$.

The null hypothesis is that there is no difference between the mean transit times on these two forms of treatment. Thus it is *not* disproved. We may therefore say that there is no convincing evidence of a difference between these two methods of administering this preparation of bran.

The second case of a paired comparison to consider is when two samples are chosen, and each member of sample 1 is paired with each of sample 2. Treatment A is then applied to all members of sample 1 and treatment B to all members of sample 2. The data are analysed in the same way as above for a single sample with paired treatments, but some thought needs to be given to the composition of the pairs.

Since the aim is to test the difference, if any, between two types of treatment, the choice of members for each pair is designed to make them as alike as possible. The more alike they are, the more apparent will be any differences due to treatment, since these will not be confused with differences in the results due to disparities between each member of the pair. The likeness within the pairs applies to attributes relating to the study in question. For instance, in a test of a drug for reducing blood pressure the colour of the patients' eyes would probably be irrelevant, but their resting diastolic blood pressure could well provide one basis for selecting the pairs. Another (and perhaps related) basis is the prognosis for the disease in patients; in general, patients with a similar prognosis are best paired. Whatever criteria are chosen, it is essential that the pairs are constructed before the treatment is given, for the pairing must be uninfluenced by knowledge of the effects of treatment.

Exercise 7.1. In 22 patients with an unusual liver disease the plasma alkaline phosphatase was found in a certain laboratory to have a mean value of 39 King-Armstrong units, standard deviation 3·4 units. What are the 95% confidence limits within which the mean of the population of such cases whose specimens come to the same laboratory may be expected to lie? *Answer:* 37·5 and 40·5.

Exercise 7.2. In Dr Pink's 18 patients the mean level of plasma phosphate was 1·7 mmol/l, standard deviation 0·8. If the mean level in the general population is taken as 1·2 mmol/l, what is the significance of the difference between that mean and the mean in Dr Pink's patients? *Answer:* $t = 2 \cdot 652, 0 \cdot 02 > P > 0 \cdot 01$.

Exercise 7.3. In two wards for elderly women in a geriatric hospital the following levels of haemoglobin were found: Ward A: 12·2, 11·1, 14·0, 11·3, 10·8, 12·5, 12·2, 11·9, 13·6, 12·7, 13·4, 13·7 g/dl; Ward B: 11·9, 10·7, 12·3, 13·9, 11·1, 11·2, 13·3, 11·4, 12·0, 11·1 g/dl. What is the difference between the mean levels in the two wards, and what is its significance? *Answer:* 0·56 g/dl; $t = $ 1·243, DF = 20, 0·5 > P > 0·1.

Exercise 7.4. A new treatment for varicose ulcer is compared with a standard treatment on 10 matched pairs of patients by measuring the number of days from start of treatment to healing of ulcer. One doctor is responsible for treatment and a second doctor assesses healing without knowing which treatment each patient had. On the standard treatment the following treatment times were recorded as numbers of days: 35, 104, 27, 53, 72, 64, 97, 121, 86, 41; and on the new treatment the following: 27, 52, 46, 33, 37, 82, 51, 92, 68, 62. What are the mean difference in the healing time, the value of t, the degrees of freedom, and the probability? *Answer:* 15 days, $t = $ 1·758, DF = 9, 0·5 > P > 0·1.

8. The x^2 tests

The distribution of a discrete variable in a sample often needs to be compared with the distribution of a discrete variable in another sample.

For example, over a period of two years Dr Gold has classified by socio-economic class the women aged 20–64 admitted to his unit suffering from self-poisoning—sample A. At the same time he has likewise classified the women of similar age admitted to a gastro-enterological unit in the same hospital—sample B. He has employed the Registrar General's five socio-economic classes, and generally classified the woman by reference to her father's or husband's occupation. The results are set out in table 8.1.

The problem Dr Gold wants to investigate is whether the distribution of the patients by social class differed in these two units. He therefore erects the null hypothesis that there is no difference between the two distributions. This is what he tests by chi-square (χ^2).

It is important to emphasise here that χ^2 tests may be carried out for this purpose only on the *actual numbers* of occurrences, *not* on percentages, proportions, means of observations, or other derived statistics. (There are some quite different purposes for which the χ^2 distribution is used, but they do not concern us here.)

The χ^2 test is carried out in the following steps:

For each observed number (O) in the table find an "expected" number (E); this procedure is discussed below.

Subtract each expected number from each observed
number   ..   ..   O − E

Square the difference   ..   .. $(O - E)^2$

Divide the squares so obtained for each cell of the
table by the expected number for that cell   .. $(O - E)^2/E$

χ^2 is the sum of $(O - E)^2/E$.

To calculate the expected number for each cell of the table consider the null hypothesis. In this case it is that the numbers in each cell are proportionately the same in sample A as in sample B. We therefore construct a parallel table in which the proportions are exactly the same for sample A as for sample B. This is done in columns (2) and (3) of table 8.2. The proportions are obtained from the totals column in table 8.1 and they are then applied to the totals row. For instance, in table 8.2, col (2), 11·80 = (22 ÷ 289) × 155; 24·67 = (46 ÷ 289) ×

155; and so on. Likewise in column (3) $10.20 = (22 \div 289) \times 134$; $21.33 = (46 \div 289) \times 134$; and so on.

Thus by simple proportions from the totals we find an expected number to match each observed number. The sum of the expected numbers for each sample must equal the sum of the observed numbers for each sample, which is a useful check. We now subtract each expected number from its corresponding observed number. The results are given in columns (4) and (5) of table 8.2. Here two points may be noted.

TABLE 8.1—*Distribution by socio-economic class of patients admitted to self-poisoning (sample A) and gastroenterological (sample B) units*

Socio-economic class	Samples		Total
	A	B	
I	17	5	22
II	25	21	46
III	39	34	73
IV	42	49	91
V	32	25	57
Total	155	134	289

The sum of these differences always equals o in each column, and each difference for sample A is matched by the same figure, but with opposite sign, for sample B. Again these are useful checks.

Then the figures in columns (4) and (5) are each squared and divided by the corresponding expected numbers in columns (2) and (3). The results are given in columns (6) and (7) of table 8.2. Finally these results, $(O - E)^2/E$, are added. The sum of them is χ^2.

A helpful technical procedure in calculating the expected numbers may be noted here. Most electronic calculators allow successive multiplication by a constant multiplier to be carried out by a short-cut of

TABLE 8.2—*Calculation of chi-square on figures in table 8.1*

Class (1)	Expected numbers		O–E		$(O–E)^2/E$	
	A (2)	B (3)	A (4)	B (5)	A (6)	B (7)
I	11·80	10·20	5·20	— 5·20	2·292	2·651
II	24·67	21·33	0·33	— 0·33	0·004	0·005
III	39·15	33·85	— 0·15	0·15	0·001	0·001
IV	48·81	42·19	— 6·81	6·81	0·950	1·009
V	30·57	26·43	1·43	— 1·43	0·067	0·077
Total	155·00	134·00	o	o	3·314	3·833

$\chi^2 = 3.314 + 3.833 = 7.147.$ DF = 4. $0.50 > P > 0.10$.

some kind. To calculate the expected numbers a constant multiplier for each sample is obtained by dividing the total of the sample by the grand total for both the samples. In table 8.1 for sample A this is $155 \div 289 = 0.5363$. . . . This fraction is then successively multiplied by 22, 46, 73, 91, and 57. For sample B the fraction is $134 \div 289 = 0.4636$. . . . This too is successively multiplied by 22, 46, 73, 91, and 57. The results are in table 8.2, columns (2) and (3).

Having obtained a value for $\chi^2 = \Sigma\{(O - E)^2/E\}$ we look up in a table of χ^2 distribution the probability attached to it. Just as with the t table, we must enter the χ^2 table at a certain number of degrees of freedom. To ascertain these requires some care.

When a comparison is made between one sample and another, as in table 8.1, a simple rule for the degrees of freedom is that they equal (number of columns minus 1) $\times$ (number of rows minus 1). For Dr Gold's data in table 8.1 this rule gives $(2 - 1) \times (5 - 1) = 4$. Another way of looking at this is to ask what is the minimum number of figures that must be supplied in table 8.1, *in addition* to all the totals, to allow us to complete the whole table. Four numbers disposed anyhow in samples A and B provided they are in separate rows will suffice.

An abbreviated version of the χ^2 table is given in table C (Appendix). Entering this at 4 degrees of freedom and reading along the row we find that Dr Gold's value of χ^2, 7.147, lies between 3.357 and 7.779. The corresponding probability is: $0.50 > P > 0.10$. This is well above the conventionally significant level of 0.05, or 5%. So the null hypothesis is *not* disproved. It is therefore quite conceivable that in the distribution of the patients between socio-economic classes the population from which sample A was drawn did not differ significantly from the population from which sample B was drawn.

QUICK METHOD

The above method of calculating χ^2 illustrates the nature of the statistic clearly and is often used in practice. But a quicker method devised by Snedecor and Irwin (1933) is particularly suitable for use with electronic calculators.

The data are set out as in table 8.1. Take the left-hand column of figures (sample A) and call each observation a. Their total, which is 155, is then Σa.

Let p = the proportion formed when each observation a is divided by the corresponding figure in the Total column. Thus here p in turn equals 17/22, 25/46. . . . 32/57.

Let $\bar{p}$ = the proportion formed when the total of the observations in the left-hand column, Σa, is divided by the total of all the observations.

Here $\bar{p} = 155/289$. Let $\bar{q} = 1 - \bar{p}$, which is the same as $134/289$. Then

$$\chi^2 = \frac{\Sigma pa - \bar{p}\Sigma a}{\bar{p}\,\bar{q}}.$$

Working with the figures in table 8.1, we use this formula on an electronic calculator in the following way:

Calculate $\dfrac{17^2}{22}$ and store in memory

,, $\dfrac{25^2}{46}$,, ,, ,, ,,

,, $\dfrac{39^2}{73}$,, ,, ,, ,,

,, $\dfrac{42^2}{91}$,, ,, ,, ,,

,, $\dfrac{32^2}{57}$,, ,, ,, ,,

,, $\dfrac{155^2}{289}$ and subtract from memory.

Withdraw result from memory on to display screen = $1 \cdot 776975$.

We now have to divide this by $\bar{p} \times \bar{q}$. Here $\bar{p} = \dfrac{155}{289}$ and $\bar{q} = \dfrac{134}{289}$.

So instead of dividing by these fractions we turn them upside down and multiply by them. Thus without removing $1 \cdot 776975$ from the display screen we carry out the following:

$$1 \cdot 776975 \times \frac{289}{155} \times \frac{289}{134}.$$

This gives us $\chi^2 = 7 \cdot 146$.

The calculation naturally gives the same result if the figures for sample B are used instead of those for sample A.

Owing to rounding off of numbers the two methods for calculating χ^2 may lead to insignificantly different results.

FOURFOLD TABLES

A special form of the χ^2 test is particularly common in practice and quick to calculate. It is applicable when the results of an investigation can be set out in a so-called "fourfold table" or "2 × 2 contingency table".

For example, Dr White, who had been inquiring into the blood pressures of the printers and sheep farmers in her general practice (p 19), believed that their wives should be encouraged to breast-feed their babies. She has records for her practice going back over 10 years in which she has noted whether the mother breast-fed the baby for at least three months or not, and these records show whether the husband was a printer or sheep farmer (or some other occupation less well represented in her practice). The figures from her records are set out in table 8.3. The disparity seems considerable, for, while 28% of the printers' wives breast-fed their babies for three months or more, as many as 45% of the farmers' wives did so. What is its significance?

TABLE 8.3—*Numbers of wives of printers and farmers who breast-fed their babies for less than three months or for three months or more*

	Breast-fed for		Total
	Up to 3 months	3 months or more	
Printers' wives	36	14	50
Farmers' wives	30	25	55
Total	66	39	105

Again the null hypothesis is set up that there is no difference between printers' wives and farmers' wives in the period for which they breast-fed their babies. The χ^2 test on a fourfold table may be carried out by a formula that provides a short-cut to the conclusion. If a, b, c, and d are the numbers in the cells of the fourfold table as shown,

			Total
	a	b	$a + b$
	c	d	$c + d$
Total	$a + c$	$b + d$	$a + b + c + d$

χ^2 is calculated from the following formula:

$$\frac{(a\,d - b\,c)^2\,(a + b + c + d)}{(a + b)\,(c + d)\,(b + d)\,(a + c)}.$$

With a fourfold table there is 1 degree of freedom in accordance with the rule given on p 45, (number of columns minus 1) × (number of rows minus 1).

Since many electronic calculators have a capacity limited to eight digits, it is advisable not to do all the multiplication or all the division in one series of operations, lest the number become too big for the display. A suitable method is as follows:

Multiply a by d and store in memory

Multiply b by c and subtract from memory

Extract difference from memory to display ..   .. $a\,d - b\,c$

Square the difference   ..   .. $(a\,d - b\,c)^2$

Divide by $a + b$ ..   .. $\dfrac{(a\,d - b\,c)^2}{a + b}$

Divide by $c + d$ ..   ..   .. $\dfrac{(a\,d - b\,c)^2}{(a + b)\,(c + d)}$

Multiply by $a + b + c + d$ .. $\dfrac{(a\,d - b\,c)^2\,(a + b + c + d)}{(a + b)\,(c + d)}$

Divide by $b + d$ ..   .. $\dfrac{(a\,d - b\,c)^2\,(a + b + c + d)}{(a + b)\,(c + d)\,(b + d)}$

Divide by $a + c$ ..   ..   .. $\dfrac{(a\,d - b\,c)^2\,(a + b + c + d)}{(a + b)\,(c + d)\,(b + d)\,(a + c)}$

With Dr White's figures we have

$$\frac{\{(36 \times 25) - (30 \times 14)\}^2 \times 105}{66 \times 39 \times 55 \times 50} = 3\cdot418.$$

Entering the χ^2 table with 1 degree of freedom we read along the row and find that $3\cdot418$ lies between $2\cdot706$ and $3\cdot841$. Therefore $0\cdot1 > P > 0\cdot05$. So, despite an apparently considerable difference between the printers' wives and the farmers' wives breast-feeding their babies for three months or more, the probability of its occurring by chance is more than 5%.

It should be emphasised again that the χ^2 test is done on the actual numbers of cases, not on, for example, percentages. But suppose the percentages are tested: do we get the same result?

For example, 28% of printers' wives and 45% of farmers' wives breast-fed their babies for three months or more. The difference is 17%. What is the standard error of this difference? It is calculated by the first method set out in Chapter 6. With Dr White's figures we have

$$\text{SE diff } \% = \sqrt{\frac{62\cdot86 \times 37\cdot14}{50} + \frac{62\cdot86 \times 37\cdot14}{55}} = 9\cdot44.$$

The difference divided by its standard error is $17/9\cdot44 = 1\cdot80$. This just falls short of the $1\cdot96$ standard errors at the 5% level of probability. Reference to table A shows that it lies between $1\cdot645$ and $1\cdot96$, corresponding to $0\cdot1 > P > 0\cdot05$, the same as with the χ^2 test.

SMALL NUMBERS

Experts differ somewhat on how small the numbers in contingency tables may be for a χ^2 test to yield an acceptable result. The following recommendations by Cochran (1954) may be regarded as a sound guide. In fourfold tables a χ^2 test is inappropriate if the total of the table is less than 20, or if the total lies between 20 and 40 and the smallest expected (not observed) value is less than 5; in contingency tables with more than 1 degree of freedom it is inappropriate if more than about one-fifth of the cells have expected values less than 5 or any cell an expected value of less than 1.

When the values in a fourfold table are fairly small a "correction for continuity" devised by Yates (1934) should be applied. While there is no precise rule defining the circumstances in which to use Yates's correction, a common practice is to incorporate it into χ^2 calculations on tables with a total of under 100 or with any cell containing a value less than 10. Armitage (1971) goes so far as to say that "it is probably wise practice to apply it for almost all χ^2 tests for 2 × 2 tables". The χ^2 test on a fourfold table is then modified as follows:

$$\frac{\{(|a\,d - b\,c|) - \frac{1}{2}(a + b + c + d)\}^2\,(a + b + c + d)}{(a + b)\,(c + d)\,(b + d)\,(a + c)}.$$

The vertical bars on either side of $a\,d - b\,c$ mean that the smaller of those two products is taken from the larger. Half the total of the four values is then subtracted from that difference to provide Yates's correction. The effect of the correction is always to reduce the value of χ^2.

Applying it to the figures in table 8.3 gives the following result:

$$\frac{\{(36 \times 25) - (30 \times 14) - (105 \div 2)\}^2 \times 105}{66 \times 39 \times 55 \times 50} = 2 \cdot 711.$$

In this case $\chi^2 = 2 \cdot 711$ falls within the same range of P values as the $\chi^2 = 3 \cdot 418$ we got without Yates's correction, $0 \cdot 1 > P > 0 \cdot 05$, but the P value is closer to $0 \cdot 1$ than it was in the previous calculation. In fourfold tables containing lower frequencies than table 8.3 the reduction in P value by Yates's correction may be of considerable significance.

FIT OF CLASS TO SAMPLE

Earlier in this chapter we compared two samples by the χ^2 test to answer the question: Are the distributions of the members of these two samples between five classes significantly different? Another way of putting this is to ask, Does each sample fit the classes in the same sort of way? A converse approach that is sometimes useful is to ask, Does each class fit the sample in the same sort of way?

For example, Dr Scarlet is an industrial medical officer of a large factory whose employees want to be immunised against influenza. Five vaccines of various types based on the current viruses are available, but nobody knows which is preferable to another. Dr Scarlet finds that 1350 employees agree to be immunised with one of the vaccines in the first week of December, so he divides the total up into five approximately equal groups. Disparities occur between their total numbers owing to the layout of the factory complex. In the first week of the following March he examines the records he has been keeping to see how many employees got influenza and how many did not. These records are classified by the type of vaccine (table 8.4).

TABLE 8.4—*People who did or did not get influenza after inoculation with one of five vaccines*

Type of vaccine	Numbers of employees		
	Got influenza	Avoided influenza	Total
I	43	237	280
II	52	198	250
III	25	245	270
IV	48	212	260
V	57	233	290
Total	225	1125	1350

In table 8.5 the figures are analysed by the χ^2 test. For this we have to determine what are the expected values. Dr Scarlet's null hypothesis is that there is no difference between the vaccines in their efficacy against influenza. We therefore assume the proportion of employees contracting influenza is the same for each vaccine as it is for all combined. This proportion is derived from the total who got influenza, and is 225/1350. To find the expected number in each vaccine group

TABLE 8.5—*Calculation of χ^2 on figures in table 8.4*

Type of vaccine	Expected numbers		O – E		$(O - E)^2/E$	
	Got influenza	Avoided influenza	Got influenza	Avoided influenza	Got influenza	Avoided influenza
I	46·7	233·3	— 3·7	3·7	0·293	0·059
II	41·7	208·3	10·3	— 10·3	2·544	0·509
III	45·0	225·0	— 20·0	20·0	8·889	1·778
IV	43·3	216·7	4·7	— 4·7	0·510	0·102
V	48·3	241·7	8·7	— 8·7	1·567	0·313
Total	225·0	1125·0	0	0	13·803	2·761

$\chi^2 = 16·564.$ DF = 4. $0·01 > P > 0·001.$

who contracted the disease we multiply the actual numbers in the "Total" column of table 8.4 by this proportion. Thus $280 \times (225 \div 1350) = 46.7$; $250 \times (225 \div 1350) = 41.7$; and so on. Likewise the proportion who did not get influenza is $1125/1350$. Again the expected numbers are calculated in the same way from the totals in table 8.4, so that $280 \times (1125 \div 1350) = 233.3$; $250 \times (1125 \div 1350) = 208.3$; and so on. The procedure is thus the same as shown in tables 8.1 and 8.2.

The calculations in table 8.5 show that χ^2 with 4 degrees of freedom is 16.564, and $0.01 > P > 0.001$. This is a highly significant result. But what does it mean?

SPLITTING OF χ^2

Inspection of table 8.5 shows that much the largest contribution to the total χ^2 comes from the figures for vaccine III. They are 8.889 and 1.778, which together equal 10.667. If this figure is subtracted from the total χ^2, $16.564 - 10.667 = 5.897$. This gives an approximate figure for χ^2 for the remainder of the table with 3 degrees of freedom (by removing the vaccine III now we have reduced the table to 4 rows and 2 columns). We then find that $0.5 > P > 0.1$, a non-significant result. But this is only a rough approximation. To check it exactly we apply the χ^2 test to the figures in table 8.4 minus the row giving those for vaccine III. In other words, the test is now performed on the figures for vaccines I, II, IV, and V. On these figures $\chi^2 = 2.983$, DF $= 3$, $0.5 > P > 0.1$. Thus the probability falls within the same broad limits as by the approximate short cut given above. We can conclude that the figures for vaccine III are responsible for the highly significant result of the total χ^2 of 16.564.

But this is not quite the end of the story. Before concluding from these figures that vaccine III is superior to the others we ought to carry out a check on other possible explanations for the disparity. The process of randomisation in the choice of the persons to receive each of the vaccines should on the average have balanced out any differences between the groups, but some may have remained by chance. The sort of questions worth examining now are: Were the people receiving vaccine III as likely to be exposed to infection as those receiving the other vaccines? Could they have had a higher level of immunity from previous infection? Were they of comparable socio-economic status? Of similar age on average? Were the sexes comparably distributed? Though these characteristics should have been more or less equalised when the groups were chosen in the first place, it is as well to check that they have in fact been equalised before attributing the numerical discrepancy in the results to the potency of the vaccine.

THEORETICAL DISTRIBUTION

In the cases so far discussed the observed values in one sample have been compared with the observed values in another. But sometimes we want to compare the observed values in one sample with a theoretical distribution.

For example, Dr Orange has a breeding population of mice in his laboratory. Some are entirely white, some have a small patch of brown hairs on the skin, and others have a large patch. According to the genetic theory for the inheritance of these coloured patches of hair the population of mice should include 51·0% entirely white, 40·8% with a small brown patch, and 8·2% with a large brown patch. In fact among the 784 mice in Dr Orange's laboratory the numbers are 380 entirely white, 330 with a small brown patch, and 74 with a large brown patch. Do the proportions differ from those theoretically expected?

The data are set out in table 8·6. The expected numbers are calculated by applying the theoretical proportions to Dr Orange's total, namely 0·510 × 784, 0·408 × 784, and 0·082 × 784. Thereafter the procedure

TABLE 8.6—*Calculation of* χ^2 *from comparison between actual distribution and theoretical distribution*

Mice	Observed cases	Theoretical proportions	Expected cases	O–E	(O–E)²/E
Entirely white	380	0·510	400	— 20	1·0000
Small brown patch	330	0·408	320	10	0·3125
Large brown patch	74	0·082	64	10	1·5625
Total	784	1·000	784	0	2·8750

$\chi^2 = 2\cdot875.$ DF = 2. $0\cdot30 > P > 0\cdot20.$

is the same as in previous calculations of χ^2. In this case it comes to 2·875. The χ^2 table is entered at 2 degrees of freedom. We find that $0\cdot30 > P > 0\cdot20$. Consequently the null hypothesis of no difference between the observed distribution and the theoretically expected one is *not* disproved. Dr Orange's data do not depart significantly from the expected frequencies.

Exercise 8.1. In a trial of a new drug against a standard drug for the treatment of depression the new drug caused some improvement in 56% of 73 patients and the standard drug some improvement in 41% of 70 patients. The results were assessed in five categories as follows: New treatment: much improved 18, improved 23, unchanged 15, worse 9, much worse 8; standard treatment: much improved 12, improved 17, unchanged 19, worse 13, much worse 9. What is χ^2 on this distribution; how many degrees of freedom are there; what is the value of P? *Answer:* 3·295; 4; P > 0·5.

8. The χ^2 tests

Exercise 8.2. An outbreak of pediculosis capitis is being investigated in a girls' school containing 291 pupils. Of 130 children who live in a nearby housing estate 18 were infested and of 161 who live elsewhere 37 were infested. What is the χ^2 value of the difference, and what is its significance? *Answer:* $\chi^2 = 3\cdot916$; $0\cdot05 > P > 0\cdot02$.

Exercise 8.3. The 55 affected girls were divided into two groups of 29 and 26. The first group received a standard local application and the second group a new local application. The efficacy of each was measured by clearance of the infestation after one application. By this measure the standard application failed in 10 cases and the new application in 5. What is the χ^2 value of the difference (with Yates's correction), and what is its significance? *Answer:* $\chi^2 = 0\cdot931; 0\cdot50 > P > 0\cdot10$.

Exercise 8.4. The construction of a reservoir several years ago in an African country brought bilharzia to four villages that stand near it. Measures taken by special teams from each village to eliminate the snails were only partially effective, and a survey in these villages gave the following figures for residual cases of bilharzia (with village population in parentheses): village A, 14 (103); village B, 11 (92); village C, 39 (166); village D, 31 (221). What are the χ^2 and P values for the distribution of the cases in these villages? Do they suggest that any one village has significantly more cases than the others? *Answer:* $\chi^2 = 8\cdot949, DF = 3, 0\cdot05 > P > 0\cdot02$. Yes, village C; if this is omitted the remaining villages give $\chi^2 = 0\cdot241, DF = 2, P > 0\cdot5$. (Both χ^2 tests by quick method.)

9. Exact probability test

Sometimes in a comparison of the frequency of observations in a fourfold table the numbers are too small for a χ^2 test (Chapter 8). The exact probability test devised by R A Fisher, J O Irwin, and F Yates (see Armitage, 1971) provides a way out of the difficulty. Tables based on it have been published—for example by Geigy (Diem and Lentner, 1970)—showing levels at which the null hypothesis can be rejected. The method itself will be described here, because with the aid of a calculator the exact probability is easily computed.

Consider the following circumstances. Some soldiers are being trained as parachutists. One rather windy afternoon 55 practice jumps take place at two localities, dropping zone A and dropping zone B. Out of 15 men who jump at dropping zone A 5 suffer sprained ankles, and out of 40 who jump at dropping zone B 2 suffer this injury. The casualty rate at dropping zone A seems unduly high, so the medical officer in charge, Captain Maroon of the Royal Army Medical Corps, decides to investigate the disparity. Is it a difference that might be expected by chance? If not it deserves deeper study. The figures are set out in table 9.1. Captain Maroon works on the null hypothesis that there is no significant difference in the proportion of injured men at each dropping zone.

TABLE 9.1—*Numbers of men injured and uninjured in parachute training at two dropping zones*

	Injured	Uninjured	Total
Dropping zone A	5	10	15
Dropping zone B	2	38	40
Total	7	48	55

The method to be described tests the exact probability of observing the particular set of frequencies in the table if the marginal totals are kept at their present values. But to the probability of getting this particular set of frequencies we have to add the probability of getting a set of frequencies showing a greater disparity between the two dropping zones. This is because we are concerned to know the probability not only of the observed figures but of the more extreme cases also.

For convenience of computation the table is changed round to get the smallest number in the top left-hand cell. We therefore begin by constructing table 9.2 from table 9.1 by transposing the upper and lower rows.

TABLE 9.2—*Numbers in table 9.1 rearranged for exact probability test*

	Injured	Uninjured	Total
Dropping zone B	2	38	40
Dropping zone A	5	10	15
Total	7	48	55

The number of possible tables with these marginal totals is 8, that is, the smallest marginal total plus 1. The 8 sets are illustrated in table 9.3. They are numbered in accordance with the top left-hand cell. The figures in our example appear in set 2.

For the general case we can use the following notation (from Armitage, 1971):

$$\begin{array}{cc|c} a & b & r_1 \\ c & d & r_2 \\ \hline s_1 & s_2 & N \end{array}$$

The exact probability for any given table is now determined from the following formula:

$$\frac{r_1!\, r_2!\, s_1!\, s_2!}{N!\, a!\, b!\, c!\, d!}$$

The exclamation mark denotes "factorial" and means successive multiplication by cardinal numbers in descending series, that is, $4!$ means $4 \times 3 \times 2 \times 1$. By convention $0! = 1$. Logarithms may be needed to handle the numbers, and a useful table of log factorials is given in Fisher and Yates (1974). But generally the factorials can be cancelled out for easy computation on a calculator (see below).

With this formula we have to find the probability attached to the observations in table 9.1, which is equivalent to table 9.2, which is denoted by set 2 in table 9.3. We also have to find the probabilities attached to the more extreme cases from set 2 back to set 0 in table 9.3.

TABLE 9.3—*Sets of frequencies in table 9.2 with same marginal totals*

0	40	40		1	39	40	
7	8	15		6	9	15	
7	48	55		7	48	55	
	Set 0				Set 1		
2	38	40		3	37	40	
5	10	15		4	11	15	
7	48	55		7	48	55	
	Set 2				Set 3		
4	36	40		5	35	40	
3	12	15		2	13	15	
7	48	55		7	48	55	
	Set 4				Set 5		
6	34	40		7	33	40	
1	14	15		0	15	15	
7	48	55		7	48	55	
	Set 6				Set 7		

The best way of doing this is to start with set 0. Call the probability attached to this set P_0. Then, applying the formula, we get:

$$P_0 = \frac{40!}{55!} \frac{15!}{0!} \frac{7!}{40!} \frac{48!}{7!} \frac{}{8!}$$

This cancels down to

$$P_0 = \frac{15!}{55!} \frac{48!}{8!}$$

For computation on a calculator the factorials can be cancelled out further by removing 8! from 15! and 48! from 55! to give

$$\frac{15 \times 14 \times 13 \times 12 \times 11 \times 10 \times 9}{55 \times 54 \times 53 \times 52 \times 51 \times 50 \times 49}.$$

We now start from the left and divide and multiply alternately. However, on an 8-digit calculator we would thereby obtain the result 0·0000317. This does not give enough significant figures. Consequently we first multiply the 15 by 1000. Alternate dividing and multiplying then gives 0·0317107. We continue to work with this figure, which is $P_0 \times 1000$, and we now enter it in the memory while also retaining it on the display.

Remembering that we are now working with units 1000 times larger than the real units, to calculate the probability for set 1 we take the value of P_0, multiply it by b and c from set 0, and divide it by a and d from set 1. That is,

$$P_1 = P_0 \times \frac{b_0 \times c_0}{a_1 \times d_1} = 0·0317107 \times \frac{40 \times 7}{1 \times 9} = 0·9865551.$$

The figure for P_1 is added into the memory and also retained on the display.

Likewise to calculate the probability for set 2 we proceed as follows:

$$P_2 = P_1 \times \frac{b_1 \times c_1}{a_2 \times d_2} = 0·9865551 \times \frac{39 \times 6}{2 \times 10} = 11·542694.$$

This too is added into the memory.

We now recall from the memory the sum contained in it, namely, $(P_0 + P_1 + P_2) \times 1000$. It is 12·560959. Dividing by 1000 we get 0·01256. This gives us the probability in one direction ("one-tailed" test). But since, as far as we know, the chance of either dropping zone having high casualties was equal, we assume that there is no difference between them in this respect. It has been debated whether to calculate P for both tails of the distribution curve by doubling $(P_2 + P_1 + P_0)$ or by some other method. Armitage (1971) favours doubling the first set of P values, which has the pleasant advantage of being the simpler as well as the theoretically preferable course.

Consequently the probability that the disparity in casualty rates at the two dropping zones could have arisen by chance is $2 \times 0.01256 = 0.025$. This is low enough for Captain Maroon to reject the null hypothesis and to look for the cause of the high rate at dropping zone A.

Exercise 9. Of 30 men employed in a small workshop 18 worked in one department and 12 in another department. In one year 5 of the 18 men reported sick with septic hands and of the 12 men 1 did so. What is the probability that such a large difference between the sickness rates in the two departments would have arisen by chance? *Answer:* P = 0·41 (that is, $2 \times 0·204$).

E

10. Rank sum tests

Values such as the mean and standard deviation that characterise a normal distribution are known as its parameters. Some data that we require to analyse do not conform to a normal distribution. Tests have been devised specially for situations such as this where we do not wish to make any assumption about the nature of the distribution. They are known as non-parametric tests. However, they can be applied also to normally distributed data.

WILCOXON'S RANK SUM TESTS

Wilcoxon's rank sum tests (Wilcoxon, 1945) are procedures of this kind. Examples of these tests follow, first on paired data (the signed rank test), then on unpaired data (the two-sample test). The Mann-Whitney U test has a similar approach to the problem and gives entirely equivalent results to the Wilcoxon two-sample test.

Dr Rosemary Mauve, a senior registrar in the the rheumatology clinic of a district hospital, is studying the possible benefits of a new drug for rheumatoid arthritis. Among other properties its effect on the course of the disease is measured by the concentration of a globulin fraction in the plasma. Twenty patients have been selected for trial of the new drug (treatment B) against a standard form of treatment (treatment A).

Owing to the nature of the disease and its response to treatment a cross-over trial on the same patients is thought to be unsuitable, so Dr Mauve divides the patients into two groups of 10 pairs, each member of a pair matching the other so far as possible in severity of the disease and prognosis. Again, as in the paired t test (p 38), it is essential to construct the pairs before treatment is given, because the choice of pairs must be uninfluenced by the effects of treatment. The intention of treatment is to lower the plasma concentration of this globulin. The reductions of concentration that treatment is known to cause are believed not to conform to a normal distribution. The actual results are set out in table 10.1.

In columns (2) and (3) of table 10.1 are listed the plasma concentrations of globulin fraction after treatment A and treatment B respectively. The difference between each pair is shown in col (4). The differences are then ranked in order in col (5), the smallest being given rank 1. When two or more differences are identical they are each allotted the half-way point between the ranks they would fill if distinct. This is

TABLE 10.1—*Wilcoxon test of significance of difference between results (on a plasma globulin fraction) of treating two groups of patients in matched pairs*

Pairs of patients (1)	Globulin fraction, g/l		Difference (4)	Rank (5)	Signed rank (6)
	Treatment A (2)	Treatment B (3)			
1	38	45	— 7	6½	— 6½
2	26	28	— 2	2½	— 2½
3	29	27	2	2½	2½
4	41	38	3	4	4
5	36	40	— 4	5	— 5
6	31	42	— 11	9	— 9
7	32	39	— 7	6½	— 6½
8	30	39	— 9	8	— 8
9	35	34	1	1	1
10	33	45	— 12	10	— 10

Totals: plus ranks, 7½; minus ranks, 47½.

done irrespective of the plus or minus sign. For instance, the differences of —2 (patient 2) and +2 (patient 3) fill ranks 2 and 3. Since $(2 + 3)/2 = 2\frac{1}{2}$ they are allotted rank 2½. Had there been three differences of size 2, irrespective of sign, they would have filled in this particular series of results ranks 2, 3, and 4. They would all have been allotted the halfway rank, $(2 + 4)/2 = 3$. And so on however many values are identical. The ranks are listed in col (5), and a useful check is that they must add up to the same total as $n(n + 1)/2$ patients; in this case $10(10 + 1)/2 = 55$. In column (6) the ranks are repeated from column (5), but to each is now added the sign of the difference from column (4).

The numbers representing the plus ranks and the minus ranks in column (6) are now added up separately, and only the smaller of the two totals is used. Irrespective of its sign it is referred to table D (Appendix) against the number of pairs used in the investigation. *Larger* rank totals than those in the table are *non*-significant at the levels of probability shown.

In this case Dr Mauve has 10 pairs of patients and the smaller rank total is 7½. This is *smaller* than the figure 8 against 10 pairs in table D. So the result is just *significant* at the 5% level. It is larger than the figure 3 shown for this number of pairs at the 1% level, so does not reach that level of significance.

UNPAIRED SAMPLES

A similar test developed by Wilcoxon is applicable to unpaired samples, and they need not be of equal size. As an example we can take Dr Mauve's data and treat them as though they had not been paired.

Statistics at Square One

The observations in the two samples are combined into a single series and ranked in order; but, in the ranking, the figures from one sample must be distinguished from those of the other sample—for

TABLE 10.2—*Wilcoxon test of significance of difference between results (on a plasma globulin fraction) of treating two unpaired groups of patients, figures for sample B are underlined*

Globulin fraction g/l	Rank	Globulin fraction g/l	Rank
26	1	36	11
27	2	38	12½
28	3	38	12½
29	4	39	14½
30	5	39	14½
31	6	40	16
32	7	41	17
33	8	42	18
34	9	45	19½
35	10	45	19½

Totals of ranks: sample A, 81·5; sample B, 128·5.

instance, by underlining. The date now appear as in table 10.2. To save space they have been set out in two columns, but a single ranking is done. The figures for sample B are underlined. Again the sum of the ranks is $n(n + 1)/2$.

The ranks for the two samples are now added separately, and the *smaller* total is used. It is referred to table E (Appendix), with n_1 equal to the number of observations in one sample and n_2 to the number of observations in the other sample. In this case they both equal 10. At $n_1 = 10$ and $n_2 = 10$ the upper part of the table shows the figure 78. The smaller total of Dr Mauve's ranks is 81·5. Since this is slightly *larger* than 78 it does *not* reach the 5% level of probability. The result is therefore not significant at that level. In the lower part of table E, which gives the figures for the 1% level of probability, the figure for $n_1 = 10$ and $n_2 = 10$ is 71. As expected, Dr Mauve's result is further from that than from the 5% figure of 78.

It is worth noting that the same data when paired produce a just significant result at the 5% level and when unpaired a just non-significant result. This disparity illustrates the value of pairing, when it can appropriately be done, in disclosing the existence of a difference that is obscured by lack of matching in the sources of the data. Pairing leads to greater sensitivity of the test because it eliminates some confusing variables.

The advantages of these tests based on ranking are that they can be safely used on data that are not at all normally distributed. Moreover, they are quick to carry out, and no calculator is needed. Their dis-advantages are, firstly, that they are generally not so sensitive as a t test, since they do not use so much information. Non-normally dis-tributed data can sometimes be transformed by the use of logarithms or some other method to make them normally distributed, and a t test performed on them then. Consequently the best procedure to adopt may require careful thought. Secondly, the extent and nature of the difference between two samples is often brought out more clearly by standard deviations and t tests than by non-parametric tests. The latter are simply tests at preselected levels of probability.

Exercise 10.1. A new treatment in the form of tablets for the prophylaxis of migraine has been introduced, to be taken before an impending attack. Twelve patients agree to try this remedy in addition to the usual general measures they take, subject to advice from their doctor on the taking of analgesics also. A crossover trial with identical placebo tablets is carried out over a period of eight months. The numbers of attacks experienced by each patient on, firstly, the new treatment and, secondly, the placebo were as follows: Patient (1), 4 and 2. Patient (2), 12 and 6. Patient (3), 6 and 6. Patient (4), 3 and 5. Patient (5), 15 and 9. Patient (6), 10 and 11. Patient (7), 2 and 4. Patient (8), 5 and 6. Patient (9), 11 and 3. Patient (10), 4 and 7. Patient (11), 6 and 0. Patient (12), 2 and 5. In a Wilcoxon rank sum test what is the smaller total of ranks? Is it significant at the 5% level? *Answer:* —30; no.

Exercise 10.2. Another doctor carried out a similar pilot study with this prepara-tion on 12 patients, giving the identical placebo to 10 other patients. The numbers of migraine attacks experienced by the patients over a period of six months were as follows. Group receiving new preparation: Patient (1), 8; (2), 6; (3), 0; (4), 3; (5), 14; (6), 5; (7), 11; (8), 2; (9), 1; (10), 9; (11), 12; (12), 4. Group receiving placebo: Patient (1), 7; (2), 10; (3), 4; (4), 12; (5), 2; (6), 8; (7), 8; (8), 6; (9), 0; (10), 5. In a Wilcoxon two-sample test what is the smaller total of ranks? Which sample of patients provides it? Is it significant at the 5% level? *Answer:* 116; the group on the placebo; no.

11. Correlation

When two or more series of observations are made it is often found that the observations in one series vary correspondingly with those in the other. The two may increase in parallel, for instance, or decrease in parallel, or as one goes up the other may go down proportionally. This relationship is called correlation. We would say, for example, that the height of children is on the average correlated with age. Since one increases with the other the correlation is called positive. In contrast there is a negative correlation, on the average, between the age of adults and the speed at which they run 100 metres.

The words "on the average" should be noted. In biology we rarely meet examples of perfect correlation, because the sources of the observations, living organisms and their products, vary from one to another and from time to time. Consequently, when we measure the degree of correlation between two sets of observations, we generally find that part of the relationship consists in a true correlation and part consists in random variation due to a multitude of indeterminate causes.

CORRELATION COEFFICIENT

The symbol used to denote the coefficient of correlation, as it is called, is r. The correlation to be discussed here, and to which this coefficient applies, is limited to what is called "straight line" correlation. This means that the relationship between the two variables can be expressed graphically by a straight line. Fortunately this is a common feature of correlation in biology. If a curved line is needed to express the relationship, other and more complicated measures of the correlation must be used.

The correlation coefficient is measured on a scale that varies from + 1 through 0 to − 1. Complete correlation between two variables is expressed by 1. When one variable increases as the other increases the correlation is positive; when one decreases as the other increases it is negative. Complete absence of correlation is represented by 0. Fig 11.1 gives some graphical representations of correlation.

SCATTER DIAGRAMS

When an investigator has collected two series of observations and he wants to see whether there is a relation between them, it is best to

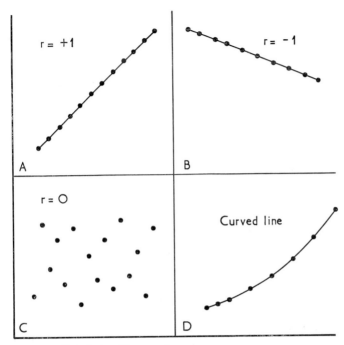

FIG 11.1—Correlation illustrated.

construct a scatter diagram first. The vertical scale represents one set of measurements and the horizontal scale the other. If one set of observations consists of experimental results and the other consists of a time scale or observed classification of some kind, it is usual to put the experimental results on the vertical axis. These represent what is called the "dependent variable". The "independent variable", such as time or height or some other observed classification, is measured along the horizontal axis, or base line.

The terms "independent" and "dependent" are apt to puzzle the beginner because it is sometimes not clear what is dependent on what. His confusion is a triumph of common sense over misleading terminology, because often enough each variable is dependent on some third variable, which may or may not be mentioned. It is reasonable, for instance, to think of the height of children as dependent on age rather than the converse. But consider a positive correlation reported by Russell *et al* (1975) between mean tar yield and nicotine yield of certain brands of cigarette. The nicotine liberated is unlikely to have its origin in the tar: probably both vary in parallel with some other factor or factors in the composition of the cigarettes. The yield of the one does not seem to be "dependent" on the other in the sense that, on the average, the height of a child depends on his age. In such cases it often does not matter which scale is put on which axis of the scatter diagram. However, if the intention is to make inferences about one variable from the other, the observations *from which* the inferences are to be made are usually put on the base line.

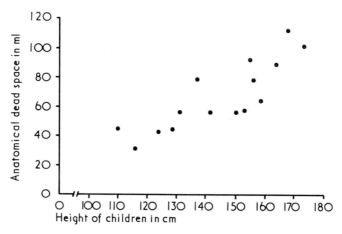

FIG 11.2—Scatter diagram of relation in 15 children between height and pulmonary anatomical dead space.

In practice the dots in a scatter diagram generally lie neither in a single straight line nor equidistant on either side of a central line but in a roughly elliptical area. For example, Kerr (1976) has shown that the "anatomical dead space" in the lungs of normal children is positively correlated with age. In other words, the older the child the larger is this space. Dr Green, a paediatric registrar, has measured the pulmonary anatomical dead space (in ml) and height (in cm) of 15 children, and prepared the scatter diagram shown in fig 11.2. Each dot represents one child, and it is placed at the point corresponding to the measurement of the height (horizontal axis) and the dead space (vertical axis). He now inspects the pattern to see whether it seems likely that the area covered by the dots centres on a straight line or whether a curved line is needed to go through its centre. In this case Dr Green decides that a straight line can adequately describe the general trend of the dots. His next step will therefore be to calculate the correlation coefficient.

CALCULATION OF CORRELATION COEFFICIENT

When making the scatter diagram (fig 11.2) to show the heights and pulmonary anatomical dead spaces in the 15 children he was studying, Dr Green set out the figures as in cols (1), (2), and (3) of table 11.1. It is helpful to arrange the observations, as he has done, in serial order of the independent variable when one of the two variables is clearly identifiable as independent. The corresponding figures for the dependent variable can then be examined in relation to the increasing series for the independent variable. In this way we get the same picture, but in numerical form, as appears in the scatter diagram.

TABLE 11.1—*Correlation between height and pulmonary anatomical dead space in 15 children*

Child number (1)	Height in cm x (2)	Dead space in ml y (3)	Col (2) squared x^2 (4)	Col (3) squared y^2 (5)	Col (2) × col (3) x y (6)
1	110	44	12 100	1 936	4 840
2	116	31	13 456	961	3 596
3	124	43	15 376	1 849	5 332
4	129	45	16 641	2 025	5 805
5	131	56	17 161	3 136	7 336
6	138	79	19 044	6 241	10 902
7	142	57	20 164	3 249	8 094
8	150	56	22 500	3 136	8 400
9	153	58	23 409	3 364	8 874
10	155	92	24 025	8 464	14 260
11	156	78	24 336	6 084	12 168
12	159	64	25 281	4 096	10 176
13	164	88	26 896	7 744	14 432
14	168	112	28 224	12 544	18 816
15	174	101	30 276	10 201	17 574
Total	2 169	1 004	318 889	75 030	150 605
Mean	144·6	66·93			

The calculation of the correlation coefficient is as follows, with x representing the values of the independent variable (in this case height) and y representing the values of the dependent variable (in this case anatomical dead space). The formula to be used is

$$r = \frac{\Sigma(x - \bar{x})\,(y - \bar{y})}{\sqrt{\Sigma(x - \bar{x})^2\,\Sigma(y - \bar{y})^2}}.$$

The computation is as follows:

Note number of observations of x   ...   .   n

Find the sum of the x observations   ...   . Σx

Find the mean of the x observations ...   .   x̄

Find the sum of the squares of the x observations   ...   ... Σx^2

Find the square of the sum of the x observations   ...   ... $(\Sigma x)^2$

Divide this by n ...   . $\dfrac{(\Sigma x)^2}{n}$

Find the sum of the squared differences of the observations from the

mean, $\Sigma(x - \bar{x})^2$, from the identity $\Sigma x^2 - \dfrac{(\Sigma x)^2}{n}$.

This procedure is exactly the same as in finding the standard deviation, except that we here stop at finding the sum of the squared
differences between the observations and their mean, $\Sigma(x - \bar{x})^2$.

The procedure is then repeated for the y observations, so that from

the identity $\Sigma(y - \bar{y})^2 = \Sigma y^2 - \dfrac{(\Sigma y)^2}{n}$ we likewise have the sum of the

squared differences of the y observations from their mean.

Multiply $\Sigma(x - \bar{x})^2$ by $\Sigma(y - \bar{y})^2$ and take
    the square toot   ...   ... $\sqrt{\Sigma(x - \bar{x})^2\,\Sigma(y - \bar{y})^2}$ (1)

This gives us the denominator of the formula.

To obtain the numerator we proceed as follows:

Multiply each value of x by the
    corresponding value of y and add
    these products together   ...   ... Σxy (2)

Multiply the sum of the x observations
    by the sum of the y observations   ... $\Sigma x \times \Sigma y$

Divide this product by the number of
    pairs of observations ...   . $(\Sigma x \times \Sigma y)/n$ (3)

Subtract (3) from (2)   ...   . $\Sigma xy - \dfrac{\Sigma x \times \Sigma y}{n}$

This is identical to $\Sigma(x - \bar{x})(y - \bar{y})$ (4)

Finally, divide (4) by (1) to give the correlation coefficient, r.

The calculations on Dr Green's data follow—see also table 11.1,
columns (4), (5), and (6). In practice the separate values for Σx^2, Σy^2,
and Σxy are not written down as they are in the table but accumulated
in the calculator to form the totals given at the foot of those columns.

$$n = 15 \qquad\qquad\qquad\qquad n = 15$$
$$\Sigma x = 2\ 169 \qquad\qquad\qquad \Sigma y = 1\ 004$$
$$\bar{x} = 144\cdot 6 \qquad\qquad\qquad \bar{y} = 66\cdot 93$$

$$\Sigma x^2 = 318\ 889 \qquad \Sigma y^2 = 75\ 030$$
$$(\Sigma x)^2/n = 313\ 637 \cdot 4 \qquad (\Sigma y)^2/n = 67\ 201 \cdot 07$$
$$\Sigma(x - \bar{x})^2 = \qquad \Sigma(y - \bar{y})^2 =$$
$$\Sigma x^2 - \frac{(\Sigma x)^2}{n} = 5\ 251 \cdot 6. \qquad \Sigma y^2 - \frac{(\Sigma y)^2}{n} = 7\ 828 \cdot 93$$
$$\Sigma xy = 150\ 605$$
$$(\Sigma x)(\Sigma y)/n = 145\ 178 \cdot 4$$
$$\Sigma(x - \bar{x})(y - \bar{y}) = \Sigma xy - \frac{(\Sigma x)(\Sigma y)}{n} = 5\ 426 \cdot 6.$$
$$r = \frac{\Sigma(x - \bar{x})(y - \bar{y})}{\sqrt{\Sigma(x - \bar{x})^2 \Sigma(y - \bar{y})^2}} = \frac{5\ 426 \cdot 6}{\sqrt{5\ 251 \cdot 6 \times 7\ 828 \cdot 93}} = 0 \cdot 846.$$

The correlation coefficient of 0·846 indicates a strong positive correlation between size of pulmonary anatomical dead space and height of child. But in interpreting correlation it is important to remember the familiar adage, *correlation is not causation*. There may or may not be a causative connection between the two correlated variables. Moreover, if there is a connection it may be indirect.

For handling large and small numbers see Chapter 13.

A part of the variation in one of the variables (as measured by its variance) can be thought of as being due to its relationship with the other variable and another part as due to undetermined (often "random") causes. The part due to the dependence of one variable on the other is measured by r^2. In Dr Green's investigation $r^2 = 0 \cdot 716$. So we can say that 72% of the variation in size of the anatomical dead space is accounted for by the height of the child.

STANDARD ERROR

The correlation coefficient also has a standard error, which for large samples is approximately $\frac{1 - r^2}{\sqrt{n}}$.

However, to test the deviation of r from 0, or nil correlation, it is better to use the *t* test in the following calculation:

$$t = r\sqrt{\frac{n - 2}{1 - r^2}}.$$

The *t* table is entered at n − 2 degrees of freedom.

For example, the correlation coefficient for Dr Green's figures was 0·846. The number of pairs of observations was 15. Applying the above formula, we have

$$t = 0 \cdot 846 \times \sqrt{\frac{15 - 2}{1 - 0 \cdot 846^2}} = 5 \cdot 72.$$

Entering the t table at $15 - 2 = 13$ degrees of freedom we find that, at $t = 5.72$, P < 0.001. So the correlation coefficient may be regarded as highly significant.

THE REGRESSION EQUATION

Correlation between two variables means that when one of them changes by a certain amount the other changes on the average by a certain amount. For instance, in Dr Green's children greater height is associated on the average with greater anatomical dead space. If y represents the dependent variable and x the independent variable, this relationship is described as the regression of y on x. The relationship can be represented by a simple equation called the regression equation. In this context "regression" (the term is a historical anomaly) simply means that the average value of y is a "function" of x, that is, it changes with x.

The regression equation representing how much y changes with any given change of x can be used to construct a *regression line* on a scatter diagram, and in the simplest case this is assumed to be a straight line. The direction in which the line slopes depends on whether the correlation is positive or negative. When the two sets of observations increase or decrease together (positive), the slope is upwards from left to right; when one set decreases as the other increases, the slope is downwards from left to right. As the line must be straight, it will probably pass through few, if any, of the dots. Apart from its being straight we have to define two other features of it if we are to place it correctly on the diagram. The first of these is its distance above the base line; the second is its slope. They are expressed in the following *regression equation:*

$$y = a + bx.$$

With this equation we can find a series of values of y, the dependent variable, that correspond to each of a series of values of x, the independent variable. The letters a and b have to be calculated from the data. The letter a signifies the distance above the base line at which the regression line cuts the vertical (y) axis. The letter b (the *regression coefficient*) signifies the amount by which a change in x must be multiplied to give the corresponding average change in y. In this way it represents the degree to which the line slopes upwards or downwards.

Once the correlation coefficient has been computed the regression coefficients are easy to work out. We use results that we have already obtained. The formulae for finding a and b are as follows (in the order in which we calculate them):

$$b = \frac{\Sigma(x - \bar{x})(y - \bar{y})}{\Sigma(x - \bar{x})^2}. \quad a = \bar{y} - b\,\bar{x}.$$

The calculation of the correlation coefficient on Dr Green's data gave the following:

$\Sigma(x - \bar{x})(y - \bar{y}) = 5\,426\cdot6$

$\Sigma(x - \bar{x})^2 = 5\,251\cdot6$

$\bar{y} = 66\cdot93$

$\bar{x} = 144\cdot6.$

Applying these figures to the formulae for the regression coefficients, we have:

$$b = \frac{5\,426\cdot6}{5\,251\cdot6} = 1\cdot033$$

$$a = 66\cdot93 - (1\cdot033 \times 144\cdot6) = -82\cdot4.$$

Therefore the equation for the regression of y on x becomes in this case

$$y = -82\cdot4 + 1\cdot033x.$$

This means that, on the average, for every increase in height of 1 cm the increase in anatomical dead space is 1·033 ml *over the range of measurements made*.

The line representing the equation is shown superimposed on the scatter diagram of Dr Green's data in fig 11.3. The way to draw the

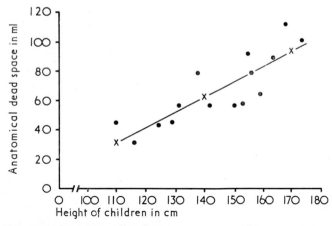

FIG 11.3—Regression line drawn on scatter diagram relating height and pulmonary anatomical dead space in 15 children (fig 11.2).

line is to take three values of x, one on the left side of the scatter diagram, one in the middle, and one on the right, and substitute these in the equation. Dr Green's figures come out as follows:

If $x = 110$, $y = (1.033 \times 110) - 82.4 = 31.2$

If $x = 140$, $y = (1.033 \times 140) - 82.4 = 62.2$

If $x = 170$, $y = (1.033 \times 170) - 82.4 = 93.2$

Though two points are enough to define the line, three are better as a check. Having put them on the scatter diagram, we simply draw the line through them.

Regression lines give us useful information about the data they are collected from. They show how one variable changes on the average with another, and they can be used to find out what one variable is likely to be when we know the other—provided we ask this question within the limits of the scatter diagram. But to project the line at either end—to extrapolate—is always risky. The relationship between x and y may change, or some kind of cut-off point may exist. For instance, a regression line might be drawn relating the chronological age of some children to their bone age, and it might be a straight line from, say, the age of 5 years to 10, but to project it up to the age of 30 would clearly lead to error.

Exercise 11.1. In a part of Kenya the incidence of kala-azar in homesteads was related to the proximity of termite hills (Southgate and Oriedo, 1962). Presumably this was because the sandfly that transmits the protozoon causing the disease found shelter there. A doctor wanting to know whether this relationship was also true for another part of Kenya visited 16 homesteads in which 40 or more people lived and for each homestead made two measurements: (1) the percentage of people suffering from kala-azar; (2) the mean distance of the five nearest termite hills. The two observations for each homestead were as follows: (1) 21%, 68 m; (2) 12%, 103 m; (3) 30%, 17 m; (4) 8%, 142 m; (5) 10%, 88 m; (6) 26%, 58 m; (7) 42%, 21 m; (8) 31%, 33 m; (9) 21%, 43 m; (10) 15%, 90 m; (11) 19%, 32 m; (12) 6%, 127 m; (13) 18%, 82 m; (14) 12%, 70 m; (15) 23%, 51 m; (16) 34%, 41 m. What is the coefficient of correlation between percentage of kala-azar cases and mean distance of termite hills? *Answer:* $r = -0.848$.

Exercise 11.2. From the data in exercise 11.1 if values of x represent mean distances of nearest five termite hills and values of y represent percentages of kala-azar cases, what is the equation for the regression of y on x? What does it mean? *Answer:* $y = 36 - 0.23x$. It means that, on the average, for every 10 m increase in mean distance of the five nearest termit hills, the percentage of cases of kala-azar falls by 2.3 ($= 10 \times 0.23$). This can be safely accepted only within the area measured here.

12. Rank Correlation

In calculating the ordinary ("product moment") correlation coefficient we worked with the actual measurements observed. Another approach is to study the order, or ranking, of the observations. For example, instead of measuring the heights of 10 men we might be able to arrange them in a line with the tallest on the right and the shortest on the left. We could then allot to each a rank numbered from 1 to 10. Furthermore, if the men ran a race we could allot a rank to each man in the order in which he finished. Thus by comparing the ranking of heights with the ranking of finishing the race we could see whether there was any connection between height and athletic success. The method by which this is done is called rank correlation.

In the circumstances of this example it would be possible, as an alternative, to calculate the product moment correlation coefficient on the measured heights of the men and the recorded times they took to complete the race. But sometimes it is virtually impossible to find measurable quantities to compare. For instance, two radiologists might be shown eight chest radiographs of cases of tuberculosis and asked to arrange them in order of severity of the disease. Differences between the radiographs might be exceedingly difficult to quantify but relatively easy for a skilled person to discern. The ranked order in which each of the radiologists placed the radiographs could be compared to show the extent to which their judgment of such matters was concordant.

Rank correlation can therefore be useful when observations are difficult or impossible to quantify exactly, and like other non-parametric methods it does not require the data to conform, even approximately, to a "normal" distribution. However, the product-moment correlation coefficient has the advantage of providing a more sensitive and generally a more reliable measure of correlation, so that if it can be used it is preferable.

The method of rank correlation described here is Kendall's. Though Spearman's is an older method and still in common use, Kendall's has both theoretical and practical advantages (Kendall, 1970). The two methods measure the data in slightly different ways, so that the coefficients derived from the same set of data usually also differ. Kendall's rank correlation coefficient is represented by the Greek letter τ (tau). Like r it varies from $+ 1$ for complete positive correlation through 0 for no correlation to $- 1$ for complete negative correlation. An example follows.

Statistics at Square One

Dr Blue is a community physician in a city where there has been much reconstruction and rehousing in recent years. The accident rate for children seemed to be surprisingly high in the newer as opposed to the older residential parts of the city. He therefore divided these into 10 districts of various sizes and ranked them, firstly, by an index of new housing and, secondly, by the children's accident rate standardised for age and sex. The results of this ranking are set out in table 12.1.

TABLE 12.1—*Ranking of 10 residential districts by (1) index of new housing and (2) standardised accident rate for children*

	District									
	A	B	C	D	E	F	G	H	I	J
Housing rank	3	9	5	10	2	7	4	8	6	1
Accident rank	1	10	2	8	3	9	4	6	7	5

To calculate the rank correlation coefficient we first rearrange the districts so that they are ranked in order for one of the attributes, housing or accidents, no matter which. They now appear as in table 12.2. The next step is to calculate two quantities P and Q on the second row (accident ranks).

TABLE 12.2—*Districts rearranged by order of rank for the rank correlation test*

	District									
	J	E	A	G	C	I	F	H	B	D
Housing rank	1	2	3	4	5	6	7	8	9	10
Accident rank	5	3	1	4	2	7	9	6	10	8

Starting with the rank on the left of the row, which is 5, we find how many ranks to its right are larger. These are ranks 7, 9, 6, 10, and 8. They make 5 ranks. We repeat this for each rank in turn to obtain the following sum:

$$P = 5 + 6 + 7 + 5 + 5 + 3 + 1 + 2 + 0 + 0 = 34$$

To calculate Q we start again with the rank at the left of the row, namely 5, and find how many ranks to the right of it are smaller. These are ranks 3, 1, 4, and 2. They add up to 4 ranks. We again repeat this process for each rank in turn to obtain the following sum:

$$Q = 4 + 2 + 0 + 1 + 0 + 1 + 2 + 0 + 1 + 0 = 11.$$

The number of districts, or *pairs* of ranks, is designated n. Then Kendall's coefficient of rank correlation is as follows:

$$\tau = \frac{P - Q}{\frac{1}{2} n (n - 1)}.$$

With Dr Blue's data we have

$$\tau = \frac{34 - 11}{\frac{1}{2} 10 (10 - 1)} = 0.51.$$

Clearly there is a considerable positive correlation between index of new housing and accident rate for children, but what is its statistical significance? (As an arithmetical check it is worth noting that in the absence of tied ranks $P + Q$ must equal $\frac{1}{2} n (n - 1)$.)

To test the significance of the correlation we consider the difference $P - Q$. Its standard error is given by

$$\sqrt{\frac{n (n - 1) (2 n + 5)}{18}}.$$

By dividing the difference by its standard error we can obtain a quantity whose statistical significance can be read from table A. But a correction for continuity is advisable, and this is made by bringing the difference of $P - Q$ 1 unit nearer to zero. Thus if $P - Q$ is positive we subtract 1 from it; if it is negative we add 1 to it. The vertical bars in the following formula indicate that, and we now calculate

$$\frac{(|P - Q| - 1)}{\sqrt{\dfrac{n (n - 1) (2 n + 5)}{18}}}.$$

Dr Blue's figures come out as follows:

$$\frac{(34 - 11) - 1}{\sqrt{\dfrac{10 (10 - 1) (20 + 5)}{18}}} = \frac{22}{11.18} = 1.968$$

This figure just exceeds 1.96 corresponding to the 5% level of probability, so the correlation coefficient of 0.51 just differs significantly from 0.

TIED RANKS

In the section on Wilcoxon's rank sum tests (p 58) we considered what to do with two or more equal ranks—that is tied ranks. These are best avoided if at all possible when calculating the rank correlation coefficient, as they are somewhat troublesome to deal with, but if they must be accepted we proceed as in the following example.

F

A headmaster of a school in the city where Dr Blue is a community physician is concerned about the possible effects of ill health on their work. He suggests to Dr Blue that a preliminary study of the problem might be appropriate. Consequently, as the academic year has just ended with final examinations Dr Blue decides to compare the examination performance of the boys in the top form with the amount of medical attention they received during the year. There are 15 boys in the form, and so he ranks them (1) by their place in the final examination, and (2) by the number of visits they paid to or received from a doctor in the year. The results are set out in table 12.3.

TABLE 12.3—*Class of 15 boys ranked by (1) order in final examination and (2) number of visits to doctor in the academic year*

	Boys														
Rank	A	B	C	D	E	F	G	H	I	J	K	L	M	N	O
Examination place	1	$2\frac{1}{2}$	$2\frac{1}{2}$	4	5	6	$7\frac{1}{2}$	$7\frac{1}{2}$	9	10	12	12	12	14	15
Medical visits	8	$5\frac{1}{2}$	2	4	2	2	$5\frac{1}{2}$	10	14	11	9	15	$12\frac{1}{2}$	7	$12\frac{1}{2}$
P	7	8	10	9	9	9	7	5	1	3	1	0	0	1	0
Q	7	3	0	2	0	0	0	2	5	2	1	2	1	0	0

$P = 70.$ $Q = 25.$ $P - Q = 45.$

Tied ranks are allotted as described in the account of Wilcoxon's rank sum tests (p 59). In the examination placing, for instance, two boys were equal in the second and third places, so each is ranked $2\frac{1}{2}$, and three were equal in the 11th, 12th, and 13th places, so each is ranked 12. As in the example with untied ranks given above the boys are ranked in order by one criterion, in this case examination place, and the rank by the other criterion, medical visits, is placed below. A modified form of the equation for the rank correlation coefficient is now calculated.

As before, P and Q are calculated on the lower row. Each rank from the left is taken in turn and the number of ranks to the right of it that are larger for P and smaller for Q is ascertained—but with this modification. When a rank in this lower row comes under a tied rank in the upper row, the other ranks beneath that tie are not compared with it.

Thus, boys B and C are tied at $2\frac{1}{2}$ in the upper row. The corresponding ranks in the lower row are $5\frac{1}{2}$ and 2. That 2 is not counted as a lower number than $5\frac{1}{2}$ when Q is calculated; it is omitted from the Q calculation for boy B. Likewise boys G and H are tied at $7\frac{1}{2}$ in the upper row. When calculating P for boy G the rank 10 of boy H under the second $7\frac{1}{2}$ is omitted. Again, boys K, L, and M are tied at rank 12 in the upper row. So when calculating P the ranks 15 and 12½ under boys L and M are not counted as being higher than the 9 for boy K; nor, in this tied group, is the rank 12½ for boy M counted as lower than 15 for boy L when calculating Q. When P and Q have been calculated by this modified procedure the difference is taken as before, P — Q.

This provides the numerator of the following equation for the rank correlation coefficient modified for use with tied ranks:

$$\tau = \frac{P - Q}{\sqrt{\{\tfrac{1}{2}n\,(n-1) - T\}}\sqrt{\{\tfrac{1}{2}n\,(n-1) - U\}}}$$

As before, n is the number of pairs of ranks, which in this case equals the number of boys. We now have to calculate T and U to take account of the ties. We do this from the following formulae:

$$T = \tfrac{1}{2}\Sigma t\,(t-1)$$
$$U = \tfrac{1}{2}\Sigma u\,(u-1).$$

Here t equals the number of ranks in each of the groups of tied ranks taken in succession in the upper row, and u equals the number of ranks in each of the groups of tied ranks taken in succession in the lower row. Thus in the upper row we have three ties, namely, 2½ and 2½, 7½ and 7½, and 12, 12, and 12. The number of ranks tied in each group is, respectively, 2, 2, and 3. We therefore write

$$\begin{aligned}
T = \ & \tfrac{1}{2} \times 2\,(2-1) + \\
& \tfrac{1}{2} \times 2\,(2-1) + \\
& \tfrac{1}{2} \times 3\,(3-1) \\
= \ & 1 + 1 + 3 = 5
\end{aligned}$$

In the lower row we also have three ties, which in order of ranking are 2, 2, and 2, 5½ and 5½, and 12½ and 12½. We therefore write

$$\begin{aligned}
U = \ & \tfrac{1}{2} \times 3\,(3-1) + \\
& \tfrac{1}{2} \times 2\,(2-1) + \\
& \tfrac{1}{2} \times 2\,(2-1) \\
= \ & 3 + 1 + 1 = 5.
\end{aligned}$$

Substituting these figures in the equation given above we have

$$\tau = \frac{45}{\sqrt{\{\tfrac{1}{2}\cdot 15\,(15-1) - 5\}}\sqrt{\{\tfrac{1}{2}\cdot 15\,(15-1) - 5\}}}$$

$$= \frac{45}{100} = 0\cdot45.$$

To test the significance of $P - Q$ and hence of τ, the formula given above for use with untied ranks gives a reasonable approximation when n is equal to or greater than 10. If n is smaller, a significance test is more complex, and Kendall (1970) should be consulted.

With Dr Blue's figures we have

$$\frac{45 - 1}{\sqrt{\dfrac{15\,(15 - 1)\,(30 + 5)}{18}}} = 2 \cdot 18.$$

From table A we find for this value of $P - Q$ divided by its standard error that $0 \cdot 05 > P > 0 \cdot 01$. Consequently these figures do suggest that there is a statistical association between place in the examination and number of visits to or from the doctor: the higher the place, the fewer the visits. Again it is important to note that a statistical association does not necessarily imply the existence of a causative connection. What it does do is to invite further study of that possibility.

Exercise 12. A dermatologist was investigating allergy to lichens among forestry workers in the north of England. He noticed that the incidence of the disease was higher among workers in forest A than in forest B. One possible reason for the difference, he thought, might be a difference in the frequency of lichen species causing the allergy. He therefore asked a botanist to select the 12 commonest species of lichen in the two forests and rank them in order of frequency in 1 km² in each forest. The botanist ranked the species as follows:

	Species											
	A	B	C	D	E	F	G	H	I	J	K	L
Forest A	1	2	3	4	5	6	7	8	9	10	11	12
Forest B	8	12	9	10	7	11	4	5	2	6	1	3

What is the rank correlation coefficient for the lichen species in these two forests ? What is its statistical significance ? *Answer:* — 0·58. 0·05 > P > 0·01.

13. Unwieldy numbers

Many electronic calculators cannot handle numbers of more than eight digits. Consequently, if the observations being studied are expressed in inconveniently large or small numbers, the numbers must be transformed to a size manageable on the calculator. This process is most commonly needed for calculating the standard deviation, and an example follows.

If the measurements of the observations are too large they can be reduced either by (1) selecting a number of convenient size and subtracting it from each measurement, or (2) selecting a number of convenient size and dividing it into each measurement. The standard deviation is then calculated on the numbers so transformed. If subtraction is done, the standard deviation on the transformed units needs no alteration, for it comes out the same as on the original units. If division is done, the standard deviation on the transformed units needs to be multiplied by the number that was chosen to divide into the original units.

TABLE F—*Standard deviation calculated on (1) original measurements of specific gravity of urine, (2) measurements from which 1000 is subtracted, (3) measurements divided by 1000*

	(1) Specific gravity	(2) − 1000	(3) ÷ 1000
	1006	6	1·006
	1008	8	1·008
	1011	11	1·011
	1016	16	1·016
	1019	19	1·019
	1021	21	1·021
	1024	24	1·024
	1025	25	1·025
n	8	8	8
Σx	8130	130	8·130
$\bar{x}$	1016·25	16·25	1·01625
Σx^2	8262480	2480	8·26248
$\Sigma(x - \bar{x})^2$	367·5	367·5	0·0003675
$\Sigma(x - \bar{x})^2/(n - 1)$	52·5	52·5	0·0000525
$\sqrt{\Sigma(x - \bar{x})^2/(n - 1)}$	7·2457	7·2457	0·0072456

The example in Table F on the specific gravity of eight samples of urine shows the principles. The measurements can in fact be accommodated on an eight digit calculator, so that the reader with such an instrument can work through the computation if he wishes. In table F, col (2), each reading of the specific gravity has 1000 subtracted from it, and in col (3) each is divided by 1000. The standard deviation at the bottom of col (2) on the measurements transformed by subtraction is the same as on the untransformed measurements in col (1). But the standard deviation at the bottom of col (3) on the measurements transformed by division needs to be multiplied by 1000 to bring it back to the original units.

If very small numbers need to be handled they can be brought to a convenient size by multiplication. For example on many calculators a series of measurements such as 0·000436 cannot be squared satisfactorily. In this case a suitable multiplier might be 1 000 000 to bring the number to 436 or 10 000 to bring it to 4·36. In either case the standard deviation is calculated on the transformed units, and the result is then divided by the number chosen to multiply the original measurements.

But numbers need not be particularly large or small to be "unwieldy" on a calculator, especially if they are close together. For example, calculation of the standard deviation of the following numbers is carried out on an 8-digit calculator: 64·22, 64·23, 64·24, 64·25, 64·27. We get $\Sigma x = 321\cdot21$, $n = 5$, $(\Sigma x)^2 = 103175\cdot86$, $(\Sigma x)^2/n = 20635\cdot172$, $\Sigma x^2 = 20635\cdot172$, $\Sigma(x - \bar{x})^2 = 0$, S.D. $= 0$. Clearly this is a useless result, because this series of numbers must have some standard deviation.

If 64 is subtracted from each number on the principle suggested above we then work with 0·22, 0·23, 0·24, 0·25, 0·27. These give $\Sigma x = 1\cdot21$, $n = 5$, $(\Sigma x)^2 = 1\cdot4641$, $(\Sigma x)^2/n = 0\cdot29282$, $\Sigma x^2 = 0\cdot2943$, $\Sigma(x - \bar{x})^2 = 0\cdot00148$, $\Sigma(x - \bar{x})^2/(n - 1) = 0\cdot00037$, S.D. $= 0\cdot0192353$. This is rounded off to 0·02.

Thus we must take care to use to best advantage the limited number of digits the calculator can show on its display panel. This is also worth bearing in mind when calculating the correlation coefficient.

Appendix

TABLE A—*Probability related to multiples of standard deviations (or standard errors) for a normal distribution*

Number of standard deviations	Probability of observation showing at least as large a deviation from the population mean
0·674	0·50
1·0	0·317
1·645	0·10
1·960	0·05
2·0	0·046
2.576	0·01
3·0	0·0027
3·291	0·001

Adapted by permission of the author and publishers from table 2.5 of *Statistical Methods in Medical Research*, by P Armitage, published by Blackwell Scientific Publications, Oxford.

TABLE B—*Distribution of* t

DF	Probability					
	0·5	0·1	0·05	0·02	0·01	0·001
1	1·000	6·314	12·706	31·821	63·657	636·619
2	0·816	2·920	4·303	6·965	9·925	31·598
3	0·765	2·353	3·182	4·541	5·841	12·941
4	0·741	2·132	2·776	3·747	4·604	8·610
5	0·727	2·015	2·571	3·365	4·032	6·859
6	0·718	1·943	2·447	3·143	3·707	5·959
7	0·711	1·895	2·365	2·998	3·499	5·405
8	0·706	1·860	2·306	2·896	3·355	5·041
9	0·703	1·833	2·262	2·821	3·250	4·781
10	0·700	1·812	2·228	2·764	3·169	4·587
11	0·697	1·796	2·201	2·718	3·106	4·437
12	0·695	1·782	2·179	2·681	3·055	4·318
13	0·694	1·771	2·160	2·650	3·012	4·221
14	0·692	1·761	2·145	2·624	2·977	4·140
15	0·691	1·753	2·131	2·602	2·947	4·073
16	0·690	1·746	2·120	2·583	2·921	4·015
17	0·689	1·740	2·110	2·567	2·898	3·965
18	0·688	1·734	2·101	2·552	2·878	3·922
19	0·688	1·729	2·093	2·539	2·861	3·883
20	0·687	1·725	2·086	2·528	2·845	3·850
21	0·686	1·721	2·080	2·518	2·831	3·819
22	0·686	1·717	2·074	2·508	2·819	3·792
23	0·685	1·714	2·069	2·500	2·807	3·767
24	0·685	1·711	2·064	2·492	2·797	3·745
25	0·684	1·708	2·060	2·485	2·787	3·725
26	0·684	1·706	2·056	2·479	2·779	3·707
27	0·684	1·703	2·052	2·473	2·771	3·690
28	0·683	1·701	2·048	2·467	2·763	3·674
29	0·683	1·699	2·045	2·462	2·756	3·659
30	0·683	1·697	2·042	2·457	2·750	3·646
40	0·681	1·684	2·021	2·423	2·704	3·551
60	0·679	1·671	2·000	2·390	2·660	3·460
120	0·677	1·658	1·980	2·358	2·617	3·373
∞	0·674	1·645	1·960	2·326	2·576	3·291

Adapted by permission of the authors and publishers from table III of Fisher and Yates: *Statistical Tables for Biological, Agricultural and Medical Research*, published by Longman Group Ltd., London (previously published by Oliver & Boyd, Edinburgh).

TABLE C—*Distribution of χ^2*

DF	Probability					
	0·50	0·10	0·05	0·02	0·01	0·001
1	0·455	2·706	3·841	5·412	6·635	10·827
2	1·386	4·605	5·991	7·824	9·210	13·815
3	2·366	6·251	7·815	9·837	11·345	16·268
4	3·357	7·779	9·488	11·668	13·277	18·465
5	4·351	9·236	11·070	13·388	15·086	20·517
6	5·348	10·645	12·592	15·033	16·812	22·457
7	6·346	12·017	14·067	16·622	18·475	24·322
8	7·344	13·362	15·507	18·168	20·090	26·125
9	8·343	14·684	16·919	19·679	21·666	27·877
10	9·342	15·987	18·307	21·161	23·209	29·588
11	10·341	17·275	19·675	22·618	24·725	31·264
12	11·340	18·549	21·026	24·054	26·217	32·909
13	12·340	19·812	22·362	25·472	27·688	34·528
14	13·339	21·064	23·685	26·873	29·141	36·123
15	14·339	22·307	24·996	28·259	30·578	37·697
16	15·338	23·542	26·296	29·633	32·000	39·252
17	16·338	24·769	27·587	30·995	33·409	40·790
18	17·338	25·989	28·869	32·346	34·805	42·312
19	18·338	27·204	30·144	33·687	36·191	43·820
20	19·337	28·412	31·410	35·020	37·566	45·315
21	20·337	29·615	32·671	36·343	38·932	46·797
22	21·337	30·813	33·924	37·659	40·289	48·268
23	22·337	32·007	35·172	38·968	41·638	49·728
24	23·337	33·196	36·415	40·270	42·980	51·179
25	24·337	34·382	37·652	41·566	44·314	52·620
26	25·336	35·563	38·885	42·856	45·642	54·052
27	26·336	36·741	40·113	44·140	46·963	55·476
28	27·336	37·916	41·337	45·419	48·278	56·893
29	28·336	39·087	42·557	46·693	49·588	58·302
30	29·336	40·256	43·773	47·962	50·892	59·703

Adapted by permission of the authors and publishers from table IV of Fisher and Yates, *Statistical Tables for Biological, Agricultural and Medical Research*, published by Longman Group Ltd., London (previously published by Oliver & Boyd, Edinburgh).

Statistics at Square One

TABLE D—*Wilcoxon test on paired samples: 5% and 1% levels of P*

Number of pairs	5% Level	1% Level
7	2	0
8	2	0
9	6	2
10	8	3
11	11	5
12	14	7
13	17	10
14	21	13
15	25	16
16	30	19

Reprinted (slightly abbreviated) by permission of the publisher from *Statistical Methods*, by George W Snedecor and William G Cochran, 6th edition (copyright), 1967, Iowa State University Press, Ames, Iowa, USA.

TABLE E—*Wilcoxon test on unpaired samples: 5% and 1% levels of P*

5% Critical points of rank sums

n_2 ↓ / n_1 →	2	3	4	5	6	7	8	9	10	11	12	13	14	15
4			10											
5		6	11	17										
6		7	12	18	26									
7		7	13	20	27	36								
8	3	8	14	21	29	38	49							
9	3	8	15	22	31	40	51	63						
10	3	9	15	23	32	42	53	65	78					
11	4	9	16	24	34	44	55	68	81	96				
12	4	10	17	26	35	46	58	71	85	99	115			
13	4	10	18	27	37	48	60	73	88	103	119	137		
14	4	11	19	28	38	50	63	76	91	106	123	141	160	
15	4	11	20	29	40	52	65	79	94	110	127	145	164	185
16	4	12	21	31	42	54	67	82	97	114	131	150	169	
17	5	12	21	32	43	56	70	84	100	117	135	154		
18	5	13	22	33	45	58	72	87	103	121	139			
19	5	13	23	34	46	60	74	90	107	124				
20	5	14	24	35	48	62	77	93	110					
21	6	14	25	37	50	64	79	95						
22	6	15	26	38	51	66	82							
23	6	15	27	39	53	68								
24	6	16	28	40	55									
25	6	16	28	42										
26	7	17	29											
27	7	17												
28	7													

1% Critical points of rank sums

n_2 ↓ / n_1 →	2	3	4	5	6	7	8	9	10	11	12	13	14	15
5				15										
6			10	16	23									
7			10	17	24	32								
8			11	17	25	34	43							
9		6	11	18	26	35	45	56						
10		6	12	19	27	37	47	58	71					
11		6	12	20	28	38	49	61	74	87				
12		7	13	21	30	40	51	63	76	90	106			
13		7	14	22	31	41	53	65	79	93	109	125		
14		7	14	22	32	43	54	67	81	96	112	129	147	
15		8	15	23	33	44	56	70	84	99	115	133	151	171
16		8	15	24	34	46	58	72	86	102	119	137	155	
17		8	16	25	36	47	60	74	89	105	122	140		
18		8	16	26	37	49	62	76	92	108	125			
19	3	9	17	27	38	50	64	78	94	111				
20	3	9	18	28	39	52	66	81	97					
21	3	9	18	29	40	53	68	83						
22	3	10	19	29	42	55	70							
23	3	10	19	30	43	57								
24	3	10	20	31	44									
25	3	11	20	32										
26	3	11	21											
27	4	11												
28	4													

n_1 and n_2 are the numbers of cases in the two groups. If the groups are unequal in size, n_1 refers to the smaller.

Reproduced by permission of the author and publisher from White, C, *Biometrics*, 1952, **8**, 33.

References

Armitage, P (1971). *Statistical Methods in Medical Research.* Oxford, Blackwell Scientific Publications.

Cochran, W G (1954). *Biometrics,* **10,** 417.

Diem, K, and Lentner, C (1970). *Documenta Geigy: Scientific Tables,* 7th edn. Macclesfield, Geigy Pharmaceuticals.

Fisher, R A, and Yates, F (1974). *Statistical Tables for Biological, Agricultural and Medical Research,* 6th edn. London, Longmans.

Hill, A B (1962). *Statistical Methods in Clinical and Preventive Medicine.* Edinburgh, Livingstone.

Hill, A B (1971). *Principles of Medical Statistics,* 9th edn. London, Lancet.

Kendall, M G (1970). *Rank Correlation Methods,* 4th edn. London, Griffin.

Kerr, A A (1976). *Thorax,* **31,** 63.

Russell, M A H, *et al.* (1975). *British Medical Journal,* **3,** 71.

Snedecor, G W, and Irwin, M R (1933). *Iowa State College of Science,* **8,** 75.

Southgate, B A, and Oriedo, B V E (1962). *Transactions of the Royal Society of Tropical Medicine and Hygiene,* **56,** 30.

Student (1908). *Biometrika,* **6,** 1.

Wilcoxon, F (1945). *Biometrics Bulletin,* **1,** 80.

Yates, F (1934). *Journal of the Royal Statistical Society,* Supplement, **1,** 217.

Index